Reiki

Discover the Ancient Healing Power of Reiki

(Unlock the Power of Palm Healing and Learn About Aura Cleansing, Developing Psychic Abilities)

Juan Maxfield

Published By **John Kembrey**

Juan Maxfield

All Rights Reserved

Reiki: Discover the Ancient Healing Power of Reiki (Unlock the Power of Palm Healing and Learn About Aura Cleansing, Developing Psychic Abilities)

ISBN   978-1-7779883-7-1

No part of this guidebook shall be reproduced in any form without permission in writing from the publisher except in the case of brief quotations embodied in critical articles or reviews.

Legal & Disclaimer

The information contained in this book is not designed to replace or take the place of any form of medicine or professional medical advice. The information in this book has been provided for educational & entertainment purposes only.

The information contained in this book has been compiled from sources deemed reliable, and it is accurate to the best of the Author's knowledge; however, the Author cannot guarantee its accuracy and validity and cannot be held liable for any errors or omissions. Changes are periodically made to this book. You must consult your doctor or get professional medical advice before using any of the suggested remedies, techniques, or information in this book.

Upon using the information contained in this book, you agree to hold harmless the Author from and against any damages, costs, and expenses, including any legal fees potentially resulting from the application of any of the information provided by this guide. This disclaimer applies to any damages or injury caused by the use and application, whether directly or indirectly, of any advice or information presented, whether for breach of contract, tort, negligence, personal injury, criminal intent, or under any other cause of action.

You agree to accept all risks of using the information presented inside this book. You need to consult a professional medical practitioner in order to ensure you are both able and healthy enough to participate in this program.

Table Of Contents

Chapter 1: Palm Healing Explained 1

Chapter 2: Starting With Meditation 19

Chapter 3: Sensing Energy, Chakras, And The Aura 38

Chapter 4: Psychic Abilities In Healing ... 83

Chapter 5: The Reiki Method 105

Chapter 6: Scanning The Aura 124

Chapter 7: Self-Healing Techniques 146

Chapter 8: Reiki 155

Chapter 9: Learning Approximately Reiki 158

Chapter 10: Negative Effects And Sides Of Reiki 161

Chapter 11: Taking Reiki Into Consideration For Health Benefits 164

Chapter 12: Reiki To Solve Problems In Life 167

Chapter 13: More Benefits Of Reiki 170

Chapter 14: Using Reiki Effectively 173

Chapter 15: Additional Treatment Advantages Of Reiki 176

Chapter 16: What To Expect From Reiki Practice 179

Chapter 17: Drawbacks Of Not Using Reiki 182

Chapter 1: Palm Healing Explained

First, we can outline and describe palm recuperation, moreover called "the laying on of fingers," which Reiki is greater normally seemed for internationally in various cultures. You will have a have a look at the information of this sort of recuperation without continually getting into Reiki genuinely however.

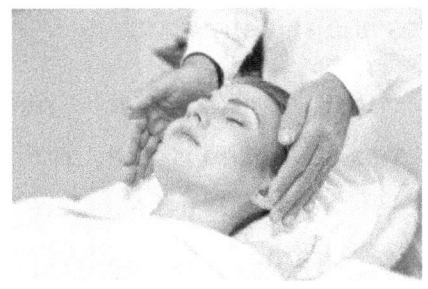

History of Palm Healing

Palm restoration has an prolonged data. Different monarchies and non secular organizations have frequently claimed excellent highbrow rights to its affords, but the critical truth is that anyone has an innate potential to heal through strength flow. Through years of evolution, the human body has developed its capacity to shield itself. For example, whilst your pores and skin gets reduce, it robotically develops a shielding layer referred to as the scab or clot. This scab protects the wound on the equal time as the pores and skin reconstructs itself underneath the scab, this is ultimately peeled away to reveal emblem-new pores and skin under it.

Another protection/recovery mechanism our body has advanced is a fever. Firstly, the presence of a fever suggests an infection inside the frame. Secondly, it starts offevolved offevolved the manufacturing of an antidote by using using triggering the immune gadget into movement to fight closer to the contamination. When your body is driven into severe conditions, it enters damage manage mode and exhibits all manner of strategies for it to hold on functioning for the duration of instances of duress.

The nice instance of this capability is the "fight or flight" reaction hardwired into each human psyche. Under annoying situations, the hypothalamus reacts and releases chemical substances into the body, which prepare it to each face the problem or run away from it. These are definitely some of the herbal abilities that our our bodies use to reply to misery.

Since the beginning of humankind and until the current, people have been making developments at an great tempo. One exception to this is inside the subject of sensory remark and the paranormal. Today, only a few rare human beings have honed their capability to acquire data with out the use of any of the 5 number one sensory inputs. Over time, humans have usually misplaced their reference to nature however have frequently received new talents and abilities.

Years in the past, we may additionally moreover need to connect with nature and energies beyond the physical realm. Before the appearance of colonization and scientific mastering, humans had a strong contact with nature, and we were quite in song with the spiritual energies of the location. This modified into vital whilst it got here to survival—on account that early humans wandered thru places searching for food and safe haven and needed to be skilled at keeping off predators and different lifestyles-threatening risks.

With the advancement of civilization, human beings have an increasing number of not noted the ones signs and instructions from nature sourced from a higher plane past this earthy realm that helped them live on in adverse environments. Humans became increasingly insensitive to the diffused indicators given off thru the earth and nature, which we even though collect sometimes through auras but conflict to recognize.

Historically talking, Master Usui, who taught Reiki, become also famous for education tenohira (palm restoration) and one-of-a-kind styles of meditation. While taking part with the naval officials of the Japanese navy, Usui started training using tenohira as an addition to first resource. Then, Hayashi Chujiro, a naval clinical professional, extended at the exquisite positions of hand placement used for modern-day palm restoration.

Hands and Our Natural Response to Pain

When we revel in ache, we right now area our fingers on that part of our body, hoping to relieve the pain. This response is based on herbal intuition. If you have were given a horrible backache, you can right now positioned your palms there with out even considering why you're doing it. Another similar reflex is blinking; we instinctively close to our eyes even as some component flies in the direction of our face.

Most would possibly say they'll be genuinely looking to make themselves experience higher via the use of the usage of massaging the ones sore spots with their arms. Another clarification is that humans have been able to heal with bioenergy because the sunrise of humankind, however only a few people can but do it in recent times. Everyone can use their fingers for restoration functions, irrespective of their age or revel in. Factors like intelligence, social reputation, ethnicity, and non secular affiliation don't have anything to do with anybody's ability to heal with their hands.

Developing the Power of Healing

When we are born, our recuperation power is mainly low, and if we do not boom it, it will live on the equal stage. If you constantly exercise your restoration electricity, it will boom in strength and live so for the rest of your lifestyles. People proficient with more bioenergy power have a extra benefit, because it will take them a shorter time to heal every one-of-a-kind individual. To start recovery, you don't need to have your recovery powers evolved to a most degree.

When you vicinity your fingers over a sore spot to heal it, healing starts offevolved offevolved right now. Even notwithstanding the fact that your initial efforts also can feel vulnerable, the results are instantaneous, no matter the truth that they may be very modest on the start. With every subsequent bypass of your hand, the go along with the waft of your bioenergy turns into more potent, and your functionality to heal receives more potent.

Just as one won't need an expertise of the criminal pointers of gravity to recognize that it exists, one does not need to understand the idea of energy healing to practice palm healing. Visiting a palm healer or an energy healer can do wonders for you—in case you go with an open mind. If you're laid low with stress, tension, or different troubles, a palm-restoration consultation will let you balance your power stages so that you can sense excellent, and in case you are already feeling proper, it's far though viable to revel in a bit bit higher. Just as we brush our hair or take a bathtub each day, cleansing your electricity frequently is also important. Sometimes human beings furthermore workout smudging or burning sage to assist put off the negativity from their energy subject on the equal time as palm healing.

Holistic Healing

Holistic recuperation consists of all of the critical equipment to assist an character find out a source of personal electricity. When we acquire private energy, we are able to dictate our mind, which shall we us bear in thoughts a better life and lets in seem it. Holistic recovery is all about locating inner peace, happiness, and experiencing whole nicely-being. Although that may appear quite philosophical and concept-scary to a layman, it is the essence of holistic healing.

In plenty much less hard terms, holistic healing is the exercise of recuperation a person whilst searching at the person as an entire and no longer truly virtually specializing of their physical symptoms. If you've got a examine the definition steady with the dictionary, holistic recovery is "characterized with the aid of manner of way of the holistic remedy of the man or woman as a whole person while considering all of the social and intellectual factors affecting them in place of focusing honestly on the signs of the disorder."

Many human beings frequently fail to find out proper comfort for his or her ailments, which forces them to start exploring other avenues of remedy, major them within the route of a holistic life-style and opportunity treatments offering treatment and healing. Often, many humans mix up holistic recovery with "alternative remedy," "integrative medication," or "complementary medicinal drug." Although all of them might not be the identical thing, what distinguishes each as separate is the focus of the treatment.

Current clinical treatment focuses on bodily signs and symptoms and signs and symptoms and signs. In holistic recovery, the healer focuses on all the factors of someone—because of this the term holistic, the goal of it's to set up a balance and concord inside the thoughts, frame, and spirit. Whether we're aware of it or no longer, life and the correct situations that it brings forth reasons us to answer to conditions in great strategies, be it bodily, mentally, spiritually, or emotionally.

Western treatment and one-of-a-kind traditional scientific practices view the frame as a separate entity from the relaxation of our being. The technique of holistic recovery perspectives the body as a reflected picture of the individual as an entire. Holistic healing does not attention on "me and my frame"; alternatively, it stresses "I am my frame." Thus, the mind and frame are a unmarried entity.

A healer needs to be aware of what the affected person is announcing, but extra importantly, what isn't being stated—"listening some of the traces"—and this information should be included into the affected man or woman's life state of affairs. Healers need to apprehend the ache or signs and symptoms and signs and symptoms of an underlying problem, whether or now not bodily or emotional. For example, if a person has insomnia because of anxiety or stress, prescribing slumbering capsules is of no want. This will simply mask the real symptoms of a deep-rooted trouble and could fail to heal their affected person.

The person have to end up pill primarily based, which, as we understand, isn't always unusual. Very quickly, the dearth of sleep leeches into one of a kind parts of the affected person's life, inflicting similarly troubles, burdening their thoughts even more. The cycle worsens, and ultimately, the individual's scenario can also deteriorate into some element even worse than it modified into first of all. In this case, the slumbering pills act as a brief-term way to an prolonged-term problem, which want to have in any other case been resolved via way of life changes and remedy.

Prana/Chi

Although Prana is more well-known as a precept of yoga, it is some thing every character has. Prana is the primordial power of the universe, which flows through our our our bodies and is dispersed through the cloth geographical regions. Steeped in Hinduism, Prana—or its Chinese counterpart, chi—is the lifestyles force or popular power. It is the amalgamation of all of the strength inside the universe, which consist of the dormant energies of nature.

It's no longer some problem that may be effects perceived as it constantly stays in a static country, diffused and immobile. Prana or chi best enters a dynamic nation even as activated with the aid of the usage of vibrations and manifests itself as magnetism, slight, warm temperature, and energy.

Prana comes from the Sanskrit word "pra," which means that ever normal, and "an," that means dynamic. The etymology of the location is "constant movement," it's related to the vibrational developments of all of the fantastic sorts of power. In Chinese, chi interprets to electricity. Thus, the complete universe is crafted from electricity and rely. Charles Darwin's Theory of Evolution suggests that all life office work originated from a unmarried not unusual supply and that the diversification and precise species tailored and advanced in response to environmental changes.

Similarly, strength is the deliver of all life forms, manifested into bear in mind, developing all of the rich contrasts and variations our international has to offer. We live within the physical realm wherein introduction is propelled by using manner of way of dualities which incorporates the necessities of yin and yang, the moon and the solar, and Shakti and Shiva. The idea of Prana is examined in contemporary technology thru Albert Einstein's Theory of Special Relativity. Einstein's idea indicates that rely and strength are the same physical entity and interchangeable. This manner that the universe is created by using strength, and we humans percent this power.

It infuses and vitalizes all types of undergo in thoughts. It furthermore merges into atoms and subatomic particles, which we already recognize are the building blocks of keep in mind wide variety and manifestations of the bodily realm. This approach that each atom, subatomic particle, and cell is an extension of Prana/chi. Experts moreover take delivery of as real with that Prana/chi has an inherent intelligence, allowing it to carry out life-preserving techniques.

What we breathe in is likewise taken into consideration to be every other shape of Prana. The physical breath corresponds to the movement of Prana into the astral backbone. Prana flows up and down this astral backbone, similar to inhalation and exhalation. The link a number of the go along with the flow of Prana and breathing patterns is the important pillar of many yoga and meditation techniques.

In Eastern treatment, chi is the crucial power flowing through the complete frame. All the organ structures are related through chi and are affected if a unmarried element is struggling, so the complete frame desires to be checked to locate the idea of the "dis – ease." The idea of Chinese treatment is that in case your body is laid low with a sickness, your chi or lifestyles stress is imbalanced, and the go with the float have to be restored. Chi and Prana are essentially the equal detail, so do now not get forced even as one is interchanged with the alternative. Acupuncture and Reiki recovery are cautiously linked with chi and repair the right glide of chi to alleviate symptoms and signs and illnesses.

Prana isn't best a trifling philosophical concept however additionally a physical substance in each enjoy. Just as electromagnetic waves and gravitational fields exist, so do the Pranic waves, fields, and chi exist within the frame regardless of the fact that we can not see them. Every single one human beings has a specific amount of Prana/chi in our our bodies, and this lifestyles strain is used for first-rate sports activities inside the course of our day and our lifetime.

When Prana is dwindled, ailments and problems creep into the body. When we have adequate chi/Prana in our body, our frame remains in fine health. When someone possesses an extra of chi/Prana, it could be transferred to other people and is used for recovery (palm healing, Reiki healing).

Without Prana, a residing being has no attention. Prana/chi is the essential building block of our holistic life. For instance, a fetus will percent its mom's Prana, and every exist as a unique entity of the overall interest earlier than the 1/three trimester. After the 1/three trimester, the developing fetus develops its non-public attention and Prana.

All the sports activities we carry out require Prana/chi—transferring, speakme, the usage of our senses, questioning, and current. A healthful man or woman also can have masses of life strain inside them, and their bodies may also additionally have a proper glide of Prana. Most illnesses, each physical or highbrow, are due to the mistaken distribution of Prana or chi due to the blockage of chakra centers and electricity channels.

The Pranic Body

In the human frame, blood is constantly flowing through our veins, capillaries, and arteries. Similarly, in our Pranic frame, Prana flows via electricity channels and pathways known as Nadis. Prana enters our frame while we breathe in. When we exercising breathing sporting sports and increase the breadth and fine of breathing, we simultaneously increase and enhance our Prana and the great of this important existence pressure. This is why respiration strategies are the form of massive a part of yoga and Pranayama.

Chapter 2: Starting With Meditation

In this bankruptcy, we are capable of examine meditation. Knowing a way to meditate effectively is vital to any kind of strength recuperation, because it locations the healer in a kingdom of calm and allows him or her to select up on unbalanced energies, song in to the receiver of restoration, and allow their own strength to go with the flow optimally. As a Reiki practitioner, you can need to meditate previous to recuperation. Here you'll analyze a few meditation physical sports you can use in the course of a Reiki consultation.

What Is Meditation?

Meditation is one of the oldest techniques of memory improvement. It includes gaining knowledge of the way to control your focus and hobby, and if you cannot, you will in no manner reap fulfillment in phrases of improving your memory. While meditating, you can need to calm your self and keep your thoughts from wandering. Classic meditation requires you to drain your mind of all thoughts and distractions. You will need a quiet spot without a outside distractions to meditate effectively. Meditation is a completely simple exercising, and all you need to do is keep the right posture and address your respiratory.

Meditation trains your mind to attention on the winning second. Relax your body, and give interest in your breath even as you keep in thoughts every inhale and exhale movement. And even as you're doing this, dissociate yourself from all your worries and regrets. However, it is simple to get distracted, however you should awareness at the triumphing second. Initially, it's tough, and you could discover yourself distracted with the resource of mind. You'll be conscious that your thoughts will constantly try to interrupt you at every opportunity. Over time, you'll be capable of empty your thoughts and recognition on the existing 2d more without problems. This is why meditation does now not artwork except you do it each day.

There are severa techniques. Each caters to precise people on a private stage. Some people reply properly to classical meditation, whilst others can also locate transcendental meditation more effective. If one form of meditation does not come up with the outcomes you want, you could attempt switching to some other shape. When people listen the word "meditation," it proper away brings up the belief of sitting nonetheless at the same time as sitting in a without a doubt uncomfortable 1/2-lotus function and chanting the phrase "ohm" again and again.

This should likely artwork for a few however may be vain for others. You want to locate what works terrific for you and preserve on with that technique. It is feasible to meditate whilst on foot, floating on water, or lying down on a hammock. It's no longer generally important a very good manner to assume uncomfortable positions and chant mantras.

Experts propose novices begin with the resource of meditating for 5 minutes. This can also additionally moreover sound like a long term to take a seat and reflect onconsideration on now not a few issue, and it is actual that even as you first start, the ones 5 mins will sense like a long time. But five minutes is the ideal amount of time for a novice. You may probable experience like giving up but persevere! Meditating for even one or minutes will can help you set up the dependancy and beef up your cognitive powers.

Meditation and Reiki

Reiki meditation is a form of meditation wherein you experience the subtle lifestyles strain power—the Prana/chi—and education it is able to offer you with large remedy. Reiki meditation includes putting your fingers on precise elements at the body and visualizing symbols that facilitate recovery memories. Reiki recuperation is one of the oldest recuperation strategies inside the international of medicine. In a international whole of horrific electricity and stress, our energy centers or chakras get blocked with the aid of the use of the impact of strain and terrible energies due to every day dwelling. Reiki intervals help with many troubles, which encompass stress and pain, and some declare they're capable of even deal with a number of the maximum extreme illnesses.

A lot of hospitals and recuperation centers provide Reiki as a supplementary remedy. If you're new to Reiki, the splendid way to start is through finding a expert practitioner and getting some shape of training or remedy instructions. Reiki meditation will help you unclog any power blockages that is probably observed to your frame and get the power flowing via it the manner it is meant to. When power begins to go along with the go with the flow thru your frame, it may help set up harmony and eliminate all of the imbalances that the ones energy blocks may additionally have created. Chakras aren't independent of each exclusive, and that they act as a whole unit. Each chakra can feature properly handiest if the possibility chakras are aligned and easy of blockages.

To energize your chakras or possibly heal them via Reiki meditation, take a seat down in a cushty role, keeping your spine upright. Take in five to 10 deep breaths and permit your body and thoughts to loosen up. You may even use chants which consist of "Om" or any mantra that appeals to you to enhance the enjoyable impact. This will relax your thoughts, so your energies are in balance.

Once you have got reached a non violent u . S . Of mind, begin meditating by means of the use of specializing within the basis chakra and little by little flow into your recognition up inside the route of the crown chakra. Placing your arms over an appropriate chakra factors can help you to decorate the recuperation effect of Reiki. Visualize the Reiki electricity coursing via your palms and coming into your body via the muse chakra.

Another manner of creating the meditation greater powerful is to visualize the colours of the respective chakra elements. For example, in case you are specializing in the root chakra, visualize the shade crimson. Keep channeling the Reiki power through your root chakra for three or four mins. Once you are performed, visualize your root chakra being bolstered and revitalized by means of the use of way of the Reiki energy and all blockages being unblocked. Repeat the same machine for all the seven chakras of your body and perform the identical manifestation to cleanse your air of thriller.

The use of restoration crystals also can intensify your Reiki meditation periods. For each chakra component, positive crystals boom the vibrational frequency of your energy. If you are looking to apply a single crystal, bypass for clean quartz, additionally known as the hold close crystal. The hold close crystal allow you to heal all of the seven chakra elements simultaneously. The use of mantras and easy music also can supplement your Reiki durations.

Reiki meditation is taken into consideration a divine gadget, and it presents an powerful way to locate answers or are seeking for steering for problems that is probably bothering you and thereby create an imbalance on your body. When you put your mind in a meditative united states, the divine strength of the universe will strive to talk with you through first rate signs and signs and symptoms and signs and logos. These messages and signs and symptoms allow you to discover the answers you're looking for, create effective adjustments internal yourself, and facilitate healing and managing issues or issues that you is probably going thru.

Remember, meditation does now not always suggest final your eyes and reciting mantras or chants. Although this may assist melt the mind and floor your self, you can adopt any technique that suits your individual. You can in truth take a seat down and stare at a candle flame, or you can be aware of calming sounds and permit your mind location out.

As with anything else, you may perform meditation every day or weekly. Trust your self on the identical time as doing it and pay attention for your intuition to choose out assets you need to attention on. For a few human beings, it is able to be easy, and for others, it would take some time to overcome the initial battle of letting skip of mind. This is in which consistency is important—the greater you exercising, the higher you can get at it. It is also important to maintain track of your progress and take a look at your improvement weekly or month-to-month.

Meditating frequently will assist you deliver best strength into your body and decorate the go with the flow of this strength via all the taken into consideration one in all a type chakras, growing a balance and making sure which you have a healthful thoughts and body at the identical time.

Benefits of Meditation

Improved Brain Activity

Improved cognition and neurological activity are some of the simplest processes of stopping the onset of neurodegenerative ailments inclusive of Alzheimer's illness and Parkinson's disease. Meditation profoundly influences reminiscence, cognition, attention, and specific mind features that commonly visit pot and degenerate with the onset of vintage age. If you meditate frequently, your later years can be spent in a much better country of fitness, with out the forgetfulness and intellectual deterioration that consists of vintage age.

Makes You Alert

Have you ever ordered a espresso with out knowing you ordered the incorrect type? And you grow to be figuring out to shop for a cappuccino while you pick an coffee? Have you again and again out of area tune of time and have been late to a dentist appointment? Or have you ever not noted your exit on the highway due to the truth you've got been distracted? These minor setbacks upload as much as making your day complex. These topics are enough to break your day and, by using extension, your mood. Meditation ensures that you are continuously aware of what's taking place around you.

Better for Mental Health

Anxiety and depression are highbrow health issues, however they'll be not due to micro organism or viruses, not like different fitness troubles. They are because of social anxiety and emotional stress. They have a horrible effect to your thoughts and first-rate of existence, appreciably lowering your existence expectancy and sturdiness if no longer handled in time. This is why the remedy of anxiety and despair is not focused upon treating one a part of the frame.

Instead, the only manner of creating development is by way of manner of enhancing the general brilliant of life via alleviating stressors that cause depression or tension. Meditation has a healthy impact on the mind and, in place of centered on one situation, continues your thoughts healthful and forestalls neurodegeneration in older people.

Tips for Better Meditation

When you meditate, pick not anything. Judging is what brings you again to the real international. Meditation calls for that you be loose to function any price to emotions, impulses, and emotions.

Keeping your attention free is the goal of the whole way. It also can be executed in small methods. As you meditate, remember what is occurring outside of your body. The surroundings in that you meditate offers you diverse sensations inside the shape of sounds, images, and smells. Learn to witness all of this without distracting your self from meditation.

The method is an critical a part of mindfulness meditation. If clean matters such as a low sound or a fly with out trouble distract you, you'll no longer attain fulfillment. Only by way of the usage of studying to disregard distractions can mindfulness meditation obtain fulfillment.

Do not surrender if you to begin with fail. It isn't the same for all of us. Some human beings find it a breeze, whilst others are without trouble distracted. The key is to preserve trying. The more you attempt, the higher you may be.

Transform your emotions. Negative feelings which include anger, infection, and jealousy can be redirected so you consider more best topics. Stand far from them, looking in silence. Watch them try to play hints in your thoughts and do no longer say a phrase.

The historical saints and ascetics of the East used meditation to live in shape, persevered the most brutal climate, and lived frugal lives. They have a look at many scriptures and recited them verbatim after the primary reading. How do you discovered it become feasible? The solution is meditation.

A go-legged feature is the first rate for meditation. The ancient sages who finished ideal happiness, additionally known as

Nirvana, felt that a bypass-legged characteristic supplied many opportunities. It is also taken into consideration the great characteristic to take your meal. This function moreover lets in you stay upright, targeted, and attentive—all the applicable conditions for a wonderful meditation.

The Biological and Neurological Effects of Meditation

Better Limbic Functions

Meditation additionally profoundly influences limbic function, verbal fluency, and could boom flexibility in cognitive capabilities. People are more and more affected by highbrow health troubles, neurodegenerative sicknesses, and character dissociation issues due to a decline in wholesome manner of existence alternatives and horrible nutritional practices.

The use of gadgets together with cellular telephones and computers also can reduce the attention span of young kids and prevent the proper improvement of the thoughts. Since maximum of the populace is desensitized inside the course of the usage of cell telephones and gadgets and is continuously being dissociated from their surroundings, this restricts the development of neurons in certain regions of the thoughts. These underdeveloped regions of the mind can lack cognitive function, growing the danger of developing neurological troubles. With the improved numbers of highbrow health problems and neurological illnesses, meditation has emerge as a powerful device this is freely available for all and sundry to apply.

Although many scientists are analyzing the manner of meditation and its results at the frame, there aren't any conclusive and definitive proofs to quantify this. In a religious context, meditation has proved to be a powerful device in growing recognition and developing spirituality. The inner peace and brilliant feelings professional after a great meditation session decorate thoughts waves to your cerebral cortex and cognitive pathways.

There have moreover been a few studies studies that investigated the consequences of meditation on abnormal growing older and neurodegeneration. Practices along with transcendental meditation and mindfulness stimulate the manufacturing of neurological connections and neurochemical receptors for your mind.

Some MRI studies have furthermore verified that the thoughts undergoes an real morphological alternate that is visible in the ones scans. It was determined that seniors who practiced meditation each day had a appreciably progressed thickness of the cerebral cortex. These neurons moreover made structural adjustments and showed an alteration in amazing regions of the mind, which encompass the advanced and inferior prefrontal cortex, the frontal cortex, the anterior cingulate cortex, and the amygdala. These regions of the mind are related to performing superb cognitive functions, which includes sensory processing, interest, limbic response, and different authorities functions.

Studies also show that each day meditation outcomes in a huge growth inner the amount of suprachiasmatic nuclei inside the hippocampus vicinity of the mind. The hippocampus is responsible for reminiscence and sensory function, and an boom in the suprachiasmatic nuclei will growth the useful functionality of the hippocampus.

The most profound effect of meditation emerge as determined in older adults. The growth in the thickness of the prefrontal cortex have come to be lots extra widespread in human beings over the age of 60, instead of their more youthful counterparts. This modified right into a robust indicator that the exercising of meditation may have a compensatory effect on neurodegeneration and showed a lower in thickness of the cerebral cortex this is introduced approximately with the useful resource of antique age. The boom within the thickness of the cerebral cortex can be attributed to numerous various factors, together with the multiplication of glial cells, neuronal arborization, and an boom inner the quantity of blood vessels in the mind. This is a sturdy argument for meditation as a way of neuroregeneration.

Chapter 3: Sensing Energy, Chakras, And The Aura

Now let us get into the priority of power. Here you will analyze more about electricity, the electricity concern, the chakra system, in addition to strength our bodies, with each defined in detail. Then we're capable of get into the priority of the air of secrecy—what it's far, how it abilities, and what it manner. Toward the surrender of this segment, we have were given furnished bodily video games on sensing energy, growing an energy ball, starting off the chakras, and seeing auras. All this understanding is vital to emerge as a healer and discover complicated areas inside the frame/aura.

The Energetic Anatomy

There are many varieties of human strength fields. They consist of the measurable magnetic and electromagnetic fields generated by using the usage of every residing cell, organ, tissue, and frame. They moreover encompass biofields which is probably subtle fields radiating from the pulsing devices of residing matters alongside side our energy our our bodies and channels.

Etheric Fields

Etheric is a word that commonly replaces air of mystery or subtle frame. Independent etheric fields are present round all vibrating devices of existence. This applies to cells, people, or maybe vegetation. A precise etheric subject is also related to your body. This term become derived from the phrase "ether"—some element that might permeate thru region at the identical time as transmitting waves of energy transversely. An etheric area surrounds the complete frame, and consequently it's far an crucial a part of someone's strength difficulty. The popular view is to take into account it a separate electricity body, and it's said to hyperlink great our our bodies to the physical body. Barbara Brennan, an expert on the air of mystery, indicates that the human energy discipline exists earlier than the increase of cells. Phoebe Bendit, a renowned creator and clairvoyant, says the identical of the auric area, and she believes that it acts as a matrix on the identical time as permeating every particle inside the body. The etheric body is related to the meridians; however, Dr. Kim Bonghan, an expert in acupuncture, shows that the ones meridians act as an interface a number of the bodily frame and the etheric strength vicinity.

Morphogenetic Fields

A morphogenetic place refers to a set of cells forming an organ or a frame shape. For example, coronary coronary coronary heart tissue is long-established from a cardiac field. In the Nineteen Eighties, Rupert Sheldrake, an English biologist, first labeled learning fields that informed the ones identified scientifically. He referred to as them morphic, active, or subtle morphogenetic fields. He additionally endorsed that an strength place is gift round and inside a morphic unit. Every residing organism belonging to a specific organization will track in to that morphic field and expand via morphic resonance. This resonance will quality take location amongst similar paperwork. This technique that a plant cannot take inside the trends of a rabbit.

Sheldrake furthermore stated the ones strength fields acted like a intellectual database. His principle explains why high quality feelings, behaviors, and other traits are handed down in a family. Many research have verified that individuals of the same species will accumulate similar conduct or tendencies even though separated, and morphogenetic fields should supply an reason behind this. His philosophy additionally stated that the morphic electricity situation of a soul ought to deliver past life recollections from one lifetime to a few special. These memories couldn't be nearby, and they might no longer be anchored in a particular life or your thoughts.

Special Energy Field

Various biofields regulate terrific emotional, religious, mental, and physical skills. The fields correspond subsequently to the unique components of the diffused body:

The physical area has the lowest frequency and regulates the bodily frame of someone.

An etheric scenario is type of a blueprint of the physical body that it surrounds. The soul has an etheric human strength location as nicely.

The emotional area regulates the emotions of the organism.

The intellectual place strategies someone's ideals, thoughts, and thoughts.

The astral situation is freed from area and time. This nexus is among the non secular and physical realm.

An etheric template lies best in a non secular location and has excessive existential beliefs.

Celestial fields act as a template for etheric fields and can get right of entry to commonplace energies.

Causal fields will direct the lower existence stages.

The Aura

For masses of years, scientists were getting to know the life of the air of mystery that surrounds every residing body. This human strength trouble has auric fields or auric layers made of bands of electricity. They be part of us to the area and surround the diffused frame. Different cultures call the charisma through way of particular names. It is referred to as an astral mild via the

Kabbalists. In Christianity, you notice it as the jewellery of slight or halos round Jesus and awesome holy figures. The human energy subject is described in a good deal extra detail in Vedic scriptures and teachings by using manner of Buddhists, Native Americans, and Rosicrucians. Pythagoras noticed it as a luminous frame and discussed this problem, too.

Since the early 1800s, there was energetic medical hobby in the thriller of the air of mystery. At the time, Jan Baptist van Helmont, a high-quality chemist and physiologist, noticed it as a few regular fluid that could permeate the whole thing. Throughout information, it has been said that the aura is considered as a few difficulty that flows and is permeable. Franz Mesmer, the founder of the check of hypnosis, recommended that a magnetic fluid charges inanimate and animate gadgets and that fabric our our our bodies may have an effect on every particular via this fluid.

Several unique homes of this strength area have been moreover decided thru Baron Wilhelm von Reichenbach. In his research as a geologist, meteorologist, and philosopher, he known as the air of thriller the Odic strain, which might possibly later be called the diffused frame. He observed that the Odic pressure had homes like an electromagnetic discipline. It has opposites or polarities, just like the electromagnetic challenge did.

In the odic subject, he understood that like draws like, on the identical time as in electromagnetism, opposites will entice each precise. Von Reichenbach moreover determined that this location may also want to drift spherical devices, convey a fee, and relate to severa colorations. According to his beliefs, the odic problem on the left half of the frame changed into a awful pole, even as the right half of changed into a incredible pole. Many other theories stated that the air of secrecy changed into flowing or fluid and consisted of many colors at the identical time as being magnetic and permeable.

For instance, in first-rate research, Dr. Walter Kilner, a clinical electrician, used colored filters and a specific kind of coal tar to examine the aura in 1911. Through this, he positioned three zones. One become a darkish layer right subsequent to a person's pores and pores and pores and skin. Another became an airy layer that turned into flowing perpendicularly to the frame. The 1/three became a delicate out of doors that had about six inches of contours.

More importantly, he determined that the charisma shifts its situation in response to the scenario's u . S . Of mind and health. Our expertise approximately this human electricity vicinity become in addition advanced with the resource of Dr. Wilhelm Reich in the early 1900s. He used experiments to test the traits of the familiar energy he called "orgone."

According to numerous metaphysicians, this organ turn out to be much like Prana or chi. Reich located strength pulsing round animate and inanimate topics inside the direction of his studies. He also placed that exchange is probably introduced approximately by way of the use of the usage of clearing regions of congestion and freeing any terrible emotional or intellectual patterns. This confirmed the relationship among bodily energies and the subtle frame, further to the connection with highbrow and emotional energies.

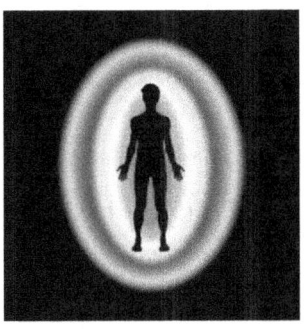

What Is the Auric Field?

We now recognize that the auric area exists, however what precisely is it? Scientists say that it's far a bio-magnetic problem surrounding the body. The felony tips of physics without a doubt united states that power fields aren't bounded. This approach that there can be no limit to how a protracted manner our bio-magnetic human energy region can make bigger. Modern device allows us to measure the coronary coronary heart's power fields up to fifteen ft in distance. This place is the maximum effective compared to others from exquisite organs. According to technological knowledge, the feature of the aura is to hold data about what takes place inside the frame instead of what takes place on the pores and skin. This is why the air of secrecy is crucial for inner health monitoring and feature.

This biomagnetic subject includes facts about each organ and tissue in the body. The currents of the coronary coronary coronary heart decide its form thinking about that this organ is the most effective. The circulatory device establishes the primary electric powered drift. The circulatory device interacts with the traumatic device, and amazing flows are created. These look like whirling styles inside the field. It isn't always viable to completely recognize the air of secrecy's reason with out gaining knowledge of about what it carries. There is still a great deal extra knowledge to be acquired regarding what the air of mystery is manufactured from.

Barbara Ann Brennan, the founding father of Brennan Healing Science and a physicist, states that the air of thriller is made of bioplasma, it is the 5th country of rely. These bioplasma particles may be subatomic and bypass in clouds. According to the philosopher Rudolf Steiner, ether is what makes up the charisma. It is an element like hole place or a negative mass. It can be surmised that the human strength vicinity is probably crafted from antimatter, permitting an power shift among worlds further to electromagnetic radiation. Thus, to deliver healing, healers should create quite a few depth inside the energies of the right right here and now to access the equal inside the anti-worlds. What is finished in a single's non-public discipline can be despatched throughout to the strength discipline of a few distinct like a message.

Brennan proposed that there are seven layers to this auric region. These layers are associated with the chakras and graduate from your frame. The seven chakras are also attuned to the diffused bodies and combine to form 3 planes. These are handy from the auric fields. She intuitively perceived degrees which is probably beyond the etheric and known as them the cosmic aircraft. These are associated with the eighth and 9th chakras. She says that the 9th has a crystalline template while the 8th is fluid.

The Auric Field and the Twelve Chakras

The twelve chakra gadget concept makes Brennan's claims approximately the 8th and 9th chakras seem legitimate. The auric fields are connected to those chakras and join what takes place internal and out of doors of the body.

The Seven Chakras

You may moreover or won't be familiar with the concept of chakras but, as a Reiki healer, you need to understand the basics about them.

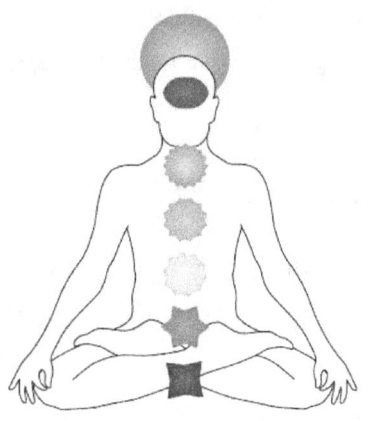

A chakra is a Sanskrit term this means that wheel. The chakras in the frame are imagined like unfastened-flowing wheels of power. There are seven chakras inside the frame, and those chakras are electricity centers. The chakras correspond to at the least one-of-a-type factors of your body and feature super functions.

Energy flows thru every chakra, and whilst they may be all open, there may be a regular glide of energy, ensuring your nicely-being. It lets in concord a number of the mind, body, and spirit. However, if one or greater of your chakras is blocked, underactive, or overactive, balance is disturbed, as a way to negatively manifest on your thoughts, body, or spirit.

Now allow us to discover approximately every chakra personally:

Muladhara or the Root Chakra

The root chakra indicates the muse of someone. It is placed at the lowest of your spine. When it is open, you could experience grounded. You will experience assured and as although you can triumph over any demanding conditions in existence. When the chakra is blocked, you will revel in insecure and unsure of your self and your abilities. The color representing this chakra is red, and the stone is hematite. The earth detail is connected to the idea chakra and practicing the Warrior 1 yoga pose will assist you open this chakra.

Image: Muladhara or Root Chakra

Svadhisthana or the Sacral Chakra

The sacral chakra is present more than one inches below your navel, within the lower belly. It controls your creativity, sexual power, and feelings. When this chakra is blocked, you could experience like you don't have any control over your lifestyles. The colour representing this chakra is orange, and the stone is a tiger's eye. The water element is attached to it, and operating toward the Bound Angle yoga pose will help you open the chakra.

Image: Svadhisthana or Sacral Chakra

Manipura or the Solar Plexus Chakra

The solar plexus chakra is the 1/3 chakra in your body, and it's far within the better belly around your stomach. This chakra controls your experience of conceitedness, self-self perception, and self confidence. Have you ever felt like there were butterflies to your stomach or maybe a pit sitting closely in it? This is because of the sun plexus chakra. When it's miles blocked, you'll doubt your self and experience overwhelming disgrace. If the chakra is open, you may be assured enough to specific your authentic self. The shade representing this chakra is yellow, and the stone is amber. The detail is hearth, and running toward the Boat Pose can be beneficial to create a free flow of electricity thru the chakra.

Image: Manipura or Solar Plexus Chakra

Anahata or the Heart Chakra

The coronary heart chakra acts as a bridge some of the better and decrease chakras on your frame. The top chakras are connected to spirituality, while the decrease chakras are associated with materiality. This chakra affects the way you get keep of or supply love. When it's far blocked, you may find out it hard to speak in confidence to people. When the coronary coronary heart chakra is open, you will be empathetic and function deep compassion for others. You will also be masses extra open to receiving love from others. The colour representing this chakra is green, and the stone is rose quartz. The air detail is connected to it, and schooling the Camel Pose in yoga will help you increase this chakra.

Image: Anahata or Heart Chakra

Vishuddha or the Throat Chakra

The throat chakra acts because the voice in your coronary heart chakra. It controls your potential to talk the reality, specific yourself, and speak with others. When the chakra is open, you may locate it clean to voice your thoughts and critiques sincerely and actually. When the throat chakra is blocked, you could discover it hard to particular what you need to mention. The coloration representing this chakra is slight blue or turquoise. The detail is sound or song. Aquamarine is the stone related to this chakra, and practicing the Fish Pose in yoga can be beneficial.

Image: Vishuddha or Throat Chakra

Ajna or the Third Eye Chakra

The further up you circulate inside the chakra device, the extra you connect with the divine. This chakra is gift among your eyes and is installed in your intuition. It will manipulate your knowledge and creativeness. This chakra can absorb information that lies past the ground. If your 0.33 eye chakra is absolutely open, you may revel in visions or have a very apt intuitive capability. The color representing this chakra is darkish blue or red, and the stone is amethyst. The detail associated with it is slight, and practising the kid's pose in yoga will help to reinforce this chakra.

Image: Ajna or Third Eye Chakra

Sahasrara or the Crown Chakra

The crown chakra lies on the crown of your head. It controls the functionality of someone to connect spiritually to the universe. It is hooked up to each internal and outer beauty. If this chakra is open, it lets in you to get proper of get entry to to a completely immoderate attention diploma. It is uncommon to find out humans who have an open crown chakra. The shade representing this chakra is violet or white, and the stone is apparent quartz. The element of divine popularity is hooked up to this chakra, and working closer to the headstand yoga pose will assist this chakra.

Image: Sahasrara or Crown Chakra

Sensing Chakras

Learning to experience chakras is a part of strength recovery as well. These strength centers are like portals in the electricity difficulty of someone. These vortices permit electricity to drift inside and from your body. The seven fundamental chakras for your body are connected to precise organs, glands, and great elements of your body. Other than the principle ones, there are different minor chakras. When there can be a disturbance within the go together with the go with the flow of electricity thru your chakras, it influences your mind, body, spirit, and life in masses of strategies. This is why power healers paintings to restore the steadiness within the strength float.

So how do you revel in chakras? Well, to begin with, it's miles less complicated to sense chakras on another man or woman in contrast to sensing chakras on yourself.

First, you want to have a vital idea of precisely wherein the chakras are placed and the way you may visualize them.

1. The root chakra is the first chakra, and it's miles gift at the base of your backbone. Think of it as a crimson wheel of energy.

2. The sacral chakra is discovered in your lower belly, and you could visualize it as an orange wheel of power.

three. The solar plexus chakra is gift amongst your navel and the bottom of your sternum in the higher belly. It can be visualized like a yellow strength wheel.

four. The coronary heart chakra lies in the center of your chest at the equal stage as your coronary heart. It is a green wheel of electricity.

5. The throat chakra is decided to your throat and may be visualized as a light blue wheel of electricity.

6. The 1/three eye chakra is present a touch above and among your eyebrows. Think of it as an indigo-colored power wheel.

7. The crown chakra is the remaining chakra and is gift at the pinnacle of your

head. It is generally related to the coloration violet or white.

Using Hands to Sense Chakras

Let us have a look at how you can sense chakras on a person the usage of your arms:

Let the character lie down on a bed or a rub down desk. Get them snug earlier than you start your Reiki session. Now keep up your palms a chunk above their body. Start transferring your fingers slowly alongside the precious channel. Begin from the place of the number one chakra till you attain the crown chakra. As you go with the flow your fingers, be conscious in case you enjoy any sensations as they pass over every chakra. Experiencing sensations together with your arms is greater common than seeing pics or colorations whilst assignment this workout. It is a specially character revel in.

When healers start training this, they generally start via sensing a few diffused energy. This can also need to show up inside the shape of heat or a humming in the hands. However, with extra revel in, strength sensitivity will increase as nicely. As you do this and enjoy the chakras, you may slowly emerge as more attuned to the electricity hobby in each chakra. Healers with more revel in will tell whilst there can be a few imbalance in a chakra. The trends of the electricity over every chakra also can range. You might possibly revel in a difference within the depth of the strength or variations in unique developments. What every healer reminiscences may be really specific from that expert thru the use of others. Do no longer worry in case you don't experience some thing; in such instances, use your imagination, and this will can help you unblock your potential to understand strength through the years. When you determined that you're feeling a few element, it is probably an energy sensation. Trust for your revel in and preserve training. Over time, your energy sensitivity will increase.

Exercises

Sensing Energy

Sensing electricity is an capability you're innately born with, but it requires exercise so you can use this capability. There isn't any specific organ within the frame that does this strength sensing. If you open your thoughts and consciousness, you can enjoy electricity. There is energy present anywhere round you and indoors you. Sensing the power internal your frame is an awful lot less complicated before the whole thing. To do that, you certainly need to begin by means of feeling your frame.

You may not have any direct enjoy running with electricity, so begin with the resource of touching the floor of your frame the use of your arms. This is the most number one way to experience your body. Another manner is with the aid of manner of growing your attention. This will will let you enjoy the body from inside. For this, you want to apply your mind to hobby on the suitable a part of the body.

As a beginner, it's far handiest to start operating collectively with your fingers as they're extra touchy to subtle shifts in energy than each exceptional a part of your anatomy.

Meditation Exercise for Sensing Energy

Keeping your decrease again right away, stand or sit consistent with your choice.

Now, bring your palms out inside the the front of your chest and preserve inches of place among them as you turn your arms towards each unique.

Now, with a relaxed thoughts, reputation all your interest for your hands and the two inches of region among them.

Take a deep breath in and flow into your hands away from every different.

Then exhale and convey your hands once more inside the route of each exclusive.

Continue this inward and outward motion together along with your arms and popularity your mind. You will sense energy inside the form of tingling, cold, warmth, power, stickiness, pressure, or lightness. All of these are energy sensations.

After doing this for a couple of minutes, slowly lower your arms lower once more to the ground. Take three breaths outside and inside.

Using this meditation, your power-sensing potential may be honed through the years. The more you increase your focus, the simpler it gets to sense power. It also can even help you increase the place of your cognizance from one single problem to the whole frame. After some time, you can revel in the electricity that surrounds your frame, the surroundings spherical you, and the energy that comes from precise humans or gadgets.

A heightened capacity to feel strength helps you to recognize the dominion of the energy to improve it. Being energy touchy may also additionally will let you get right of get entry to to lots more data, which permits you are making better picks in existence.

Creating an Energy Ball

So, what is an electricity ball, and how are you going to create one?

Have you ever felt such as you want a boost of electricity? Do you need to get higher at manifesting and be able to do it quick? Well, nowadays, you can discover ways to do that with an energy ball.

You also can have heard of a chi ball, and this is precisely what an electricity ball is. Chi is a time period used for life pressure power. With a chi ball or an strength ball, you can connect to the strength of the powerful stress of life and the universe. This will then will assist you to use the electricity actually.

Learning to make an strength ball will will assist you to use it at the same time as you want to offer yourself or someone else some excessive excellent power. It can be applied in lots of strategies:

To re-energize at the same time as you experience fatigued or exhausted.

To enjoy better whilst you are underneath the climate.

To heal your puppy after they feel sick.

To add a layer of protection spherical your self.

To occur what you want on a specific day.

Creating an power ball manner developing an strength situation internal your palms. Energy is pulled into your arms like catching a ball, and the electricity from this ball of electricity can then be harnessed. This energy may be implemented to any vicinity you need.

If you don't forget it, you will realize that you have already sensed power along side your hands. For instance, you'll probably have felt a superb way after shaking a person's hand. They would possibly make you enjoy uncomfortable, or they may deliver off warmth that makes you receive as true with them. Even whilst someone touches your arm to comfort you, you'll probable have felt the electricity of their love closer to you. When a person hugs you, it allows you to collect loving strength from their coronary heart chakra as well as their hand chakra.

Hand Chakras

There is a chakra inside the palm of every of your palms. These chakras are wheels of power that may receive and release power. Your hand chakras will help your appear creativity, openness, and self belief. When you open these chakras, you open yourself as a great deal as many stuff. You end up greater receptive inside the direction of compliments, and your self confidence gets boosted. You begin celebrating your talents and gadgets. You are extra open to debating in area of arguing with human beings. It gives you the capacity to be extra touchy to situations. Like some other chakra in the frame, your hand chakras can be overactive, blocked, or underactive. This is why it is important to learn how to keep a wholesome go with the flow of uninterrupted electricity going thru them.

Exercise

Take a deep breath in, after which allow it out. Do this a few times. Now visualize a white slight coming from your crown place and filling you with strength.

Center your self collectively with your coronary heart chakra and push the energy from there into the earth. Then visualize a golden flow into of moderate developing from the earth thru your feet into your body. Visualize this golden power starting and activating every chakra as it moves up your body. As it does this, it moves out from the top of your head and connects with the white moderate all over again.

Now visualize all the electricity from all your chakras moving towards your palms and locating an go out.

Bring your fingers together in the front of you and then rub them collectively a piece. Slowly pull your fingers some distance from every different and popularity on the way you enjoy. You can also experience a pulling sensation within the location among your hands. As you carry the palms inside the course of every unique, you may revel in a few resistance. This is the strength created via workout.

Keep pulling your arms inward and outward till you experience like a ball of energy is gift amongst them. You will feel like a actual electricity ball lies amongst your hands.

During this exercise, you may enjoy some tingling in your fingertips or your palms. You can also moreover enjoy them shake. There can be a hot or cold sensation popping out of your hands, too. While some human beings can see the energy ball, it is greater important that permits you to enjoy it.

Keep playing around with the electricity to your arms till you sense which include you simply have an electricity ball. It may additionally additionally additionally take practice, but you will quick create such electricity balls for Reiki. When you revel in like an strength ball is ready in some unspecified time in the destiny of an exercise, it may be used for healing. The ball of electricity can be directed within the route of the location of restoration. For instance, if you or a person else has a stomachache, you can direct the energy ball in the direction of that precise vicinity to sell recuperation.

Healers will instinctively inform whilst the healing manner is completed. When you experience this, in truth rub your arms together and away from every different. This allows you to launch the energy out of your palms. Do now not maintain strength in your hands after the recuperation and, more importantly, don't take in strength from someone else and maintain it to your frame.

Opening the Chakras

The chakras within the body contribute to a person's nicely-being. When the chakras are open and energetic, with a consistent go together with the drift of power going through, someone is in quality fitness. However, most parents have some chakras which might be closed, half of of-open, overactive, or underactive in the long run or each other. When this takes region, there may be a loss of balance in our structures.

To be healed and to heal a person else with Reiki, you want to open your chakras or theirs and repair the stableness. When you want to open your chakras, you do no longer ought to recognition on any overactive chakras. This excessive interest generally takes area to make up for the inaction within the chakra this is closed. When you open the closed chakra, the overactive chakra will forestall compensating for it, and the power glide might be balanced yet again.

Opening the Root Chakra

The root chakra is set up to physical focus and being comfortable in conditions. When this chakra is open, you could enjoy strong, steady, practical, and balanced. If it's miles closed, you'll experience yourself continuously mistrusting human beings and locating it difficult to be gift. On commencing the chakra, you need to revel in a deeper connection with your physical body and the prevailing.

When this chakra is underactive, it will make you annoying or worrying. You will frequently sense unwelcome spherical humans. When this chakra is overactive, you will act greedily and materialistically. You will now not be open to any changes and constantly are on the lookout for protection. To keep away from these emotions and open your chakra, you want to move—take a walk spherical a park, carry out a bit yoga, or in reality clean your home. These sports will make you aware of your body and beautify the idea chakra. Ground your self. Stand instantly but in a comfortable manner. Keep your toes apart at a shoulder-width distance and bend your knees a touch. Then waft the pelvis a bit ahead whilst balancing your body. Your weight need to enjoy evenly dispensed over your feet. Now sink this weight beforehand.

Keep your body positioned like this for a couple of minutes.

Once you floor yourself, lower your self proper right down to a bypass-legged sitting position. Place your palms over every knee and fingers grew to end up upward. Touch the suggestions of your index finger along side your thumb tips. Then popularity on the idea chakra and its significance. Visualize this chakra because it lies the various anus and the genitals. Use the sound "LAM" to chant virtually.

While doing this, loosen up on the equal time as you discovered of the chakra and what it technique in your life. Think of the manner you need the chakra to have an effect on your lifestyles. Visualize a red flower that is closed. Imagine effective energy being radiated from this flower due to the fact the petals slowly open. Holding your breath, settlement your perineum, and launch.

Opening the Sacral Chakra

The sacral chakra is attached to sexuality and feeling. When this chakra is open, your emotions may be released liberally, and you can explicit your self without feeling overemotional. You might be outgoing and passionate. It may also even ensure which you have not any problems with sexuality. When this chakra is underactive, it will reason you to be emotionless or unemotional. You will not open up resultseasily to each person round you. When this chakra is overactive, you'll be too emotional and sensitive most of the time. It also can even increase your sexual wishes.

Get down to your knees and sit with an upright again. Be comfortable. Place one give up the other and lay them to your lap. Both palms must be grew to end up upward. The right hand need to lie over the left hand. The palm of your left hand must be touching the palms of your proper hand with the thumbs gently touching as nicely.

Now region your attention on in which the sacral chakra lies near the sacral bone and don't forget what it signifies. Use the sound "VAM" to start really however silently chanting.

While you try this, be comfortable as you decided of the significance of the sacral chakra. Think of the way you want this chakra to paintings for your lifestyles. Repeat all of this till you revel in without a doubt relaxed and cleansed.

Opening the Navel Chakra

This chakra is established to self guarantee. When the chakra is open, you may enjoy like you're on top of things and dignified. When the chakra is underactive, you'll be indecisive and act passively. It will make you continuously worrying. When it's miles overactive, the chakra will make you aggressive and imperious. Get down on your knees and be comfortable. Your again want to be immediately however no longer stiff.

Place your palms in the front of you, in the front of your belly. This is a hint beneath in which the sun plexus lies. Join your arms collectively in a prayer-like hand feature however together along side your arms going via far from you. Keep your fingers straight and bypass your thumbs. Now recognition for your navel chakra and meditate on what it suggests.

The chakra is present a piece above your navel within the course of your spine. Start chanting the word "RAM" definitely however silently. Try and loosen up at the same time as you do this but maintain concentrating at the chakra. Think of techniques it presently impacts your lifestyles and the manner you want it to be. Keep repeating this until you enjoy like your chakra is cleansed and strong.

Opening the Heart Chakra

The coronary coronary coronary heart chakra is attached to love, endearment, and being involved. If the chakra is open, it will make you pleasant and compassionate. You will constantly have amicable relationships with the human beings spherical you. When it's miles underactive, you'll be unfriendly and cold. When the chakra is overactive, you may act greater lovingly than people might need you to. This form of love and care often seems to smother others, and they will see you as a selfish character. Sit down in a skip-legged characteristic. Place every give up every knee with the hands going via upward.

Touch the guidelines of your thumbs collectively at the side of your index hands. Then flow your right hand up on your chest. Hold it a piece under the lower half of of your breastbone. Now interest at the coronary coronary heart chakra gift at the level of your coronary heart within the spine. Use the word "YAM" to surely however silently chant. Try to lighten up while you try this. Think of the chakra and its importance. Think of the way you want the coronary heart chakra to effect your life. Repeat this exercise till you feel cleansed.

Opening the Throat Chakra

This chakra is attached to conversation and self-expression. If the throat chakra is open, you may discover it easy to specific your self. Art will seem like a first rate medium for self-expression. When the chakra is underactive, you'll appear like a shy man or woman to others for the cause that you may no longer talk an excessive amount of. This chakra is probably blocked if you find out your self lying too regularly. When it's far overactive, you talk an excessive amount of and annoy the human beings spherical you, and also you save you being a super listener. Get down on your knees and sit down.

Join the hands of every palms with every finger other than your thumbs crossed. Your thumbs have to be lying upward and touching on the pointers. Now start thinking about the throat chakra and its importance. The chakra is gift at the lowest of your throat. Chant the word "HAM" silently to your self. Relax as you chant and consider the which means that of this chakra. Repeat this workout for a couple of minutes until you experience intensely cleansed.

Opening the Third Eye Chakra

This chakra is set up to perception. If the 1/3 eye chakra is open, you've got many desires and will revel in clairvoyance. When it's miles underactive, you may depend upon certainly one of a type human beings to make picks and assume for you. You can be compelled most of the time and depend on ideals an excessive amount of. When the chakra is overactive, you may have a tendency to daydream too much. You may even start hallucinating even as this happens in extremes. Sit down in a cross-legged role. Bring your fingers together within the the front of the lower half of your breast.

The hints of your middle hands need to touch every specific as they factor far from you. Bend your extraordinary palms and preserve them touching on the pinnacle phalanges. Your thumbs want to fulfill on the pinnacle and element at you. Now start focusing for your 1/three eye chakra, this is gift simply above the middle of every your eyebrows. Use the word "AUM" or "OM" to begin chanting silently. Try and loosen up on the same time as you do all this and maintain concentrating on the 1/three eye chakra. Think of ways the chakra influences your lifestyles, its significance, and the manner you need it to feature. Repeat this till you revel in intensely cleansed.

Chapter 4: Psychic Abilities In Healing

While meditation and sensing energies are beneficial, it additionally allows to have a few psychic abilities, collectively with clairvoyance and clairsentience. When recuperation someone with Reiki, messages and visions have a tendency to go returned thru, which help with the healing way and/or need to be transferred to the affected individual. Here you may find out how psychic capabilities may be useful in Reiki recovery. There are physical video games that you may positioned into impact to broaden your psychic skills as well.

Regardless of your stance on psychics and psychic powers, all people has a totally specific intuition and manner of mastering and manifesting psychic skills. In truth, in line with some of the most famous psychics, each one parents possesses that otherworldly enjoy, and all we need to do is attention on it and keep studying a manner to enlarge our psychic skills. Psychic powers and "instinct" are very comparable, and they may be frequently used interchangeably.

In addition, without a doubt all people own an otherworldly experience, and the capability to tap into that strength also can mirror on our functionality to enjoy, see, and pay attention things past the physical realm and help us delve into the psychic realm. This may additionally display up every day, both knowingly and unknowingly.

Still having a difficult time being glad? Think about this: have you ever ever ever felt like a person is watching you and turned round to find someone is gazing you? Do you truly agree with that this concept popped into your mind randomly, or is there some issue more to it than meets the eye? Have you ever felt wonderful energy even as you walk right right right into a room with out even information something about the folks that is probably within the room? All of those may be looked at as random thoughts that get up on your mind. They additionally can be visible as a number of the terrific examples of the intuitive psychic present all of us very personal.

Akin to any present or capability, we're able to reactivate and hone the ones psychic capabilities to turn out to be brighter, stronger, and extra colorful variations of ourselves. It can emerge as a very practical and pretty effective tool for us, that might help us navigate through the adventure of life in unique regions, whether or not or not or no longer in our relationships, our profession paths, imaginative skills, or some component else that may be crucial to us.

To upload to those nice benefits, on the same time as you're making a conscious choice to harness your intuitive competencies, it impacts your lifestyles and creates a amazing chain response that enhances and improves the intuitive powers of the individuals who are part of your life. If this is sufficient to convince you to start the adventure of amping up your intuitive dial, it's miles now time to take a look at a number of the approaches to increase and hone your psychic competencies.

Developing Your Psychic Abilities

Be Open to the Possibility of Tapping into Your Psychic Skills

The first and vital element that inhibits someone's adventure into growing and exploring their psychic and intuitive abilities is their worry or near-mindedness closer to the undertaking available. According to maximum psychic experts, maximum humans are afraid of their herbal psychic competencies, specially because of the functionality horrible results that might encompass the enjoy. It is crucial to apprehend that these gadgets aren't a few trouble to worry.

These herbal psychic abilties have constantly been indoors us to assist lead us within the route of our maximum ability.

They act as navigational gear for us to journey via the journey of lifestyles. The first step inside the direction of developing your psychic capabilities is the clean act of being willing and open to tapping into your psychic capabilities. Without believing in yourself, almost nothing is a success. Experts advise that developing a declaration to the universe citing which you are open and prepared to discover those psychic gives is useful. This will let you prevent the concern and open your thoughts to the brighter possibilities these otherworldly sports activities can supply.

Learn to Read People's Energies

Have you ever observed how some humans supply off a totally terrible "vibe" or electricity for no concrete purpose? This isn't a few difficulty that your mind certainly concocts with none reason; rather, it is your psychic instinct coming thru. This is what "analyzing a person's energy" approach, and it's far a competencies you could amplify and beautify with time and workout. One way of doing that is via continuously tough yourself to examine and interpret humans's electricity, seeing past their facades and what they are pronouncing, and tuning into their vibes.

Although that can sound very precis, and you'll be wondering how one reads human beings's energies, it is heaps simpler than you might anticipate. Simply spending time with the man or woman is a brilliant region to begin. Doing this allows you to observe your thoughts and emotions approximately that man or woman, and the way those feelings replicate on that character is a superb manner of analyzing their energy.

According to many specialists, reading someone's energy is viable even earlier than straight away talking or interacting with them. For instance, in case you are prepared in line on the grocery store, you may faucet into the energy of the man or woman in the decrease back of you or in front of you and note what comes up in your thoughts. If it feels excessive fine, strike up a verbal exchange with them to find out whether or not your intuition changed into correct otherwise you misjudged the man or woman. It takes some time and workout before you begin analyzing humans efficiently.

Develop a Connection with Your Spirit Guides

A spirit guide is a subject that many people are skeptical approximately and is regularly frowned upon, particularly via way of folks that aren't familiar with the hassle. As individuals with instinct and psychic abilities, spirit courses are some element that we can all name directly to garner intellectual and emotional useful resource. Spirit guides may be looked at as precise and advanced soul mentors in the angelic realm and help us through guiding and training us topics that we can also normally no longer be able to.

Most professional psychics accept as real with that we also are associated with anyone close whom we can also furthermore have misplaced and who also can have crossed to the "excellent side." One of the most commonplace techniques of identifying and locating your spirit manual is via using requesting very precise signs and symptoms and signs and symptoms and symptoms from the universe. For example, if you are at the crossroads of creating a very important preference and also you want affirmation to understand which you are at the right track, you can ask for a signal from the universe via manner of requesting a few component as strange as seeing a purple panther.

The exceptional consequences come about while you get specific together together with your requests whilst requesting a signal, so on the identical time as you truly do get maintain of a signal from the universe, there can be in fact no denying that it is a sign out of your spirit publications and not honestly every extraordinary random incidence.

Communicating on the aspect of your spirit courses receives an awful lot less difficult if you do it daily. If you have not been talking on your spirit publications, there isn't thousands to worry about because of the truth it's far an entire lot much less tough than maximum human beings expect. The exceptional problem you want to do is in reality check in collectively along with your spirit guides throughout the day. It's vital to take notice of any visualizations or intuitive nudges that would come to thoughts after speakme together with your spirit guide.

Begin Predicting How Places Appear

Reading and decoding a person's power isn't the best manner to growth your psychic intuition. To broaden a well-rounded psyche, you can moreover exercise "psychic seeing," greater popularly called "clairvoyance."

Most professionals recommended education some distance off-viewing physical sports. For example, the subsequent time you're planning to transport someplace that you have in no manner visited, like a trendy restaurant, someday in advance of your real go to, near your eyes and "claim" what you want to look in that place.

Draw a rudimentary depiction of your vision on a bit of paper regardless of what comes up. When you go to the place later, you may examine your drawing to what the area really looks as if. You can also find out many similarities among what you anticipated and what you observe, and sometimes the similarities may be very unique. For instance, the location of a window or the precise form of potted flora you previously predicted at the same time as schooling clairvoyance can be present.

Exercises That Help You Develop Clairvoyance

Visualization

Visualization is a shape of workout meant to decorate a selected part of you, similar to strolling out or operating closer to yoga (which is supposed to enhance your physical attributes). Visualization can help make stronger and pleasant-music the 0.33-eye muscle companies present in your mind. The high-quality element approximately this method is that you may do this exercise the use of almost some thing.

Many humans decide on using flora (you can even use actual vegetation to make the revel in greater enticing and interactive). Start the exercising through placing a flower within the front of you and searching at it, searching for to maintain any mind from your thoughts, other than the flower. Next, near your eyes and visualize the flower with as thousands detail as you in all likelihood can.

Visualize one-of-a-kind factors of the flower, along with its shade, shape, and period. Flood your mind with those facts as efficiently as you can. Practicing those clairvoyant sports activities frequently will help you growth and hone your psychic talents.

Daydreaming

Although many people may also additionally have a first rate opinion as regards to daydreaming, a large part of clairvoyance is the functionality to visualize subjects for your thoughts. Try strolling down reminiscence lane and go through in mind the ones teenagers days at the same time as letting your logical thoughts take a lower back seat and loosen up for some time. Try to loose your thoughts from the cacophony of mind that commonly bombard your psyche and close to your eyes.

Focus on your forehead, especially on the vicinity between your eyebrows or the "1/three eye" area. Try speakme together along side your spirit publications and make a request for them to expose you peaceful and exquisite images. Avoid searching for to control your visualizations or overthinking what you're currently visualizing. Allow your mind to wander, and allow your spirit publications connect with your internal self through clairvoyance.

Setting Intentions

Once you have finished turning into acquainted together with your spirit guides, education clairvoyant sporting sports becomes thousands a lot much less complex and further comforting. Intuitive provides which encompass clairvoyance, clairaudience, claircognizance, and clairsentience are the primary techniques spirit courses talk with you, and the higher you are at communicating with them, the greater they will can help you in.

If you feel like you are in a stagnant state of thoughts, indecisive, and uncertain of what to do first, ask your spirit courses for steering. Setting the proper intentions to your existence and soliciting for divine steerage out of your spirit publications can change your life. Once you've got were given got finished placing the proper intentions in lifestyles, you need to look for the signs and symptoms that your spirit courses offer you with.

Seeing Auras

Contrary to well-known perception, auras are actual, and honestly every body can find out them. An air of thriller may be exceptional defined as a area of electricity that surrounds all dwelling creatures. For a start, you can exercise seeing auras with the resource of asking a pal to face inside the front of a sturdy-colored ground or wall. Stand lower back approximately 8 feet (stand lower back enough so that you can see them from head to toe whilst no longer having to look up or down).

Try focusing on the middle of your friend's forehead (the 1/3 eye) and visualize yourself searching through their bodily body. Gradually you may start noticing a glittery vicinity spherical their head. Voila! You have efficiently visible their air of mystery. Regular exercising will make the method easier.

Meet Other Mediums and Psychics

Being a psychic healer or Reiki healer is a totally unique profession path. There are sure barriers and traumatic situations that people who choose this career direction face—the rest of the arena will in no manner apprehend you or get what you do. The journey becomes masses simpler and extra worthwhile if you have the assist of those who recognize what you do and the challenges you face. They also can give you some beneficial hints and serve as extremely good exercise companions as a manner to extend and sharpen your competencies.

Learn How to Turn Your Gifts "ON" and "OFF"

Once you have got correctly superior your gift of clairvoyance, the subsequent component that you can want to do is to discover ways to manage it as and on the equal time as the want arises. It is crucial to show it "ON" satisfactory whilst you want to and allow pass at the same time as you want to music out of things. Prior to training any sporting activities associated with clairvoyance, begin with the smooth ritual of visualizing the act of lighting fixtures a candle inside your mind. While you're doing so, invite your spirit publications, and you may get a revel in that your gadgets have became on. This candle visualization exercise will allow your spirit courses and religious helpers provide you divine assist and boom your instinct and spiritual communicative capabilities.

Learning to show off your clairvoyant and psychic instinct is some other problem that you will need to analyze as you growth your abilties. Like turning it ON, keep in mind blowing out the candle as quickly as you've got got finished working within the path of. Once you've got wrapped the entirety up, remember blowing out the candle in your thoughts and ensuring that you pay gratitude for your non secular helpers for his or her divine guide. Doing this may assist you harness your provides and manipulate them while you are not going for walks with them or have finished any restoration or given a psychic analyzing to a purchaser.

Maintain a Journal

Once you have started out out growing a connection with your spirit courses similarly in your "higher self," you may need to write down the essential subjects that you be aware and the changes that display up after you have got were given started to grow to be extra intuitive. Many specialists take delivery of as real with that if meditation is chocolate, journaling is peanut butter. Writing down vital thoughts, intentions and manifestations let you get in touch together with your better self and spirit publications, thereby enhancing your instinct and clairvoyance.

For instance, consider the moments in existence wherein you had been immensely happy and thankful. It can be some thing from a near-loss of lifestyles enjoy to a loved one traveling suddenly. It may be some factor groundbreaking, or it may be a few aspect as clean as staying in for the weekend with your companion and having an intimate revel in with them.

Jot down the way you've got been feeling on the time and the way that revel in stayed with you and modified you within the days that accompanied. It assist you to relive those crucial moments that helped you are taking your intuition and psyche to some other degree with out forgetting the important statistics. Journaling also can be a splendid interest to interact in after a meditation consultation while the thoughts is in a relaxed and snug nation. It will assist you preserve suitable power and raise your "vibrations."

Develop Healthy Food Habits

The meals you devour makes you what you're and impacts your instinct and vibrations. Eating wholesome ingredients does now not typically suggest simplest consuming leafy greens or salads for each unmarried meal. Incorporating high vibrational meals into your regular healthy dietweight-reduction plan, which incorporates clean fruit, darkish chocolate, complete components, and getting rid of especially processed food merchandise will let you enlarge a more potent charisma and lift your lively vibe. Eating more healthful meals also permits you sense better physical, thereby making it less complicated to expand your instinct and psychic capabilities.

Activate Your Third Eye

The zero.33 eye or the pineal gland is widely considered the seat of psychic intelligence and clairvoyance and is regularly referred to in Eastern Mysticism and Egyptian statistics. The zero.33 eye works like a muscle. The more you operate it and flex it, the stronger it will become. Activating the 1/3 eye is not a complicated venture; it is pretty clean. For starters, vicinity your index finger on the 0.33 eye (the location between your eyebrows) and lightly faucet on the region some instances and recollect that it's far organising. Feeling a tingling sensation in that area is regular because it approach that your clairvoyance is getting activated. Repeat this exercise frequently, and you may begin noticing a few vital changes in your psyche and clairvoyance. If you're

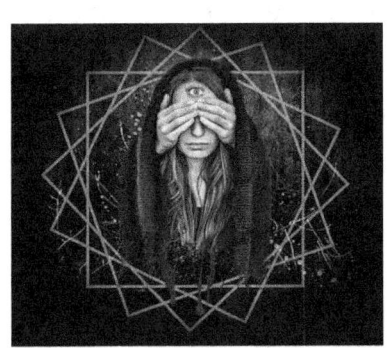

having hassle activating your zero.33 eye, you may be a part of a spiritual development circle or take specific training wherein greater skilled people who have already lengthy long gone through this technique can provide you with religious guidance and assist you set off your zero.33 eye in a stable and loving environment.

Strengthen Your Third Eye

Even despite the fact that this may be the last detail on the list, it is probably the maximum important workout which you need to engage in regularly. The 0.33 eye is the seat of all psychic capabilities and in which your clairvoyance stems from. As you hone and increase your psychic skills, you need to learn how to get hold of as genuine with them. You ought to be able to take delivery of as authentic with the visualizations and intuitive photos that are available in your mind whilst practicing recovery rituals and psychic readings. You want to often practice meditation and self-reflective strategies for you to prompt and beautify your talents. Use crystals such as fluorite and moonstone and region them on your 0.33 eye to draw strength from the crystals and guide your psychic skills and clairvoyance.

Chapter 5: The Reiki Method

A Brief History of Reiki

Although there were severa tries at explaining the data of Reiki, alas, maximum of those factors are based totally on mysticism and the real want to validate a specific form of Reiki. Most of these factors lack validated facts. Therefore, to artwork on a reality-based outlook, allow us to dig deeper into the sphere of Reiki and try to give an explanation for what it sincerely is.

Mikao Usui or Usui Sensei Is Considered via Many People to Have Been the Creator of Reiki

Usui's version of Reiki completed most effective to the handiest of a kind recovery methodologies he grow to be answerable for coming across and growing. When learning the information about the muse of Reiki, we discover that in advance than the upward thrust in recognition of Usui's Reiki methods, Reiki healing changed into practiced in Japan in four great procedures.

Most of these snippets of records come from two Japanese Reiki researchers: Toshitaka Mochitzuki Sensei and Hiroshi Doi Sensei. After the era of Usui Reiki, a Japanese therapist named Matji Kawakami got here up with a very precise fashion of Reiki recuperation referred to as Reiki Ryoho in 1919, information of which can be determined in his e-book entitled Reiki Ryoho to Sono Koka or Reiki Healing and Its Effects. The different patterns everyday have been Senshinryu Reiki Ryoho with the resource of Kogetsu Matsubara, Reikan Tonetsu Ryoho via Reikaku Ishinuki, and Seido Reisho Jitsu via using Reisen Oyama.

Although there are one-of-a-kind opinions on what must or ought to not be called Reiki, we want to don't forget that there are numerous super patterns and disciplines of Reiki restoration that have their lineage going once more to Usui Reiki. It is considered a shape of electricity that every person can use, and masses of have finished so over time. It is steady to mention that any recovery method that applies Reiki energy may be referred to as Reiki and not really those modalities described by means of way of Usui Sensei.

The Essence of Reiki

When we attention on Reiki energy for any reason—be it recovery, education, or giving attunements to your clients—specially whilst using Fire Reiki for placements and ignitions, one turns into increasingly more aware about a wealth of positivity and particular features that Reiki strength embodies.

The exceptional trends flow beyond the special states of consciousness that we are normally aware about, and Reiki energy can enhance us into transcendental stages of pleasure, happiness, and peace. In addition, the ones characteristics are also useful for human beings to expand healthful and high-quality developments as part of their personalities. Since all Reiki modalities understand loose will, none of these modalities will help us heal or cross past proper right right into a better state of mind besides we're open to it and invite it to perform that. This approach that Reiki's restoration techniques are best effective if we're inclined to alternate.

A person's potential to find out flaws and perilous private functions inside themselves and their willingness to permit them to move is of maximum importance within the event that they want to move ahead with their non-public healing and intellectual improvement. The Reiki manner can involve whatever that could help enhance the overall first rate of Reiki strength that a person can channel or imbibe and expand the traits taken into consideration healthful for a person to personal.

Some of the first-class and healthful person tendencies that Reiki can increase and boom include patience, compassion, non-competitiveness, self-love, and love for others. It takes us to an area of popularity of others' thoughts and beliefs, and it moreover enables us emerge as accepting and non-judgmental, empowering our ability to forgive others and enlarge gratitude for all the splendid matters we've skilled and are blessed with, along side buddies and family. This on my own can extensively enhance the remarkable of pleasure and peace we enjoy in existence and, most significantly, it'll boom our capability to channel the deliver of Reiki strength into an everlasting and sturdy feeling of protection that embodies all Reiki modalities.

Understanding that is what's going to ultimately will let you appreciate Reiki healing and its limitless potential. This concept is absolutely tested by way of way of the reality that maximum sensei of Reiki, collectively with Usui Sensei and Hayashi Sensei, advocated all their college college students to paintings on improving and refining the amazing of Reiki power that they have got been able to channeling. It is also very clean from the concept that if Reiki is a shape of limitless capability, as most humans will agree it's far, then irrespective of how actual and effective you're at channeling Reiki energy, it's far generally viable a terrific way to end up better and further powerful at it.

Just receiving the attunement and ignition does now not come up with whole get right of entry to to Reiki energy, however it does imply which you are able to channel Reiki power to a wonderful diploma, and if you can work further on that problem, your ability to channel a higher and extra sensitive form of strength will become an increasing number of powerful. This aspect of self-interest turns into clearer at the same time as you exercising Holy Fire Reiki as you start to revel in a fair higher stage of peace, pride, and love, and it's going to show you the way fantastic and critical it's far to embody Reiki power into your normal existence.

Benefits of Reiki Healing

Reiki is an ancient and easy recuperation technique touting some profound benefits in some unspecified time inside the destiny of the artwork of slight touch, having a immoderate notable attitude, and the switch of quality electricity. Whether you are adopting Reiki to address emotional trauma, non secular, and emotional development, or to balance your power degrees, Reiki has endless advantages. Let us observe some of the blessings that Reiki recovery may moreover result in.

It is critical to maintain in mind that Reiki does now not cause one unmarried element of the frame and as an opportunity desires the whole frame right now. The switch of splendid electricity is one of the most powerful tools for recovery the frame and mind, and this is how Reiki is effective in restoration all related factors of any bodily or intellectual scenario in desire to simplest targeting that circumstance.

Promoting Balance and Harmony

Reiki restoration adopts a completely non-invasive approach to the transfer of strength. Through this energy transfer, your frame can repair stability at some point of all of the wonderful structures of the mind, body, and spirit. This creates a balance and concord indoors you and helps you to keep most important a remarkable manner of existence.

Improves Focus and Mental Clarity

Reiki methodologies remind receivers to be gift within the second in preference to being stuck inside the beyond or worrying approximately the future. The strength transfer allows the thoughts to reputation at the prevailing second and not preserve onto beyond errors or be constantly worrying about the destiny. This allows human beings emerge as more accepting about the unsure nature of life and will help one sell high-quality reactions to massive conditions, people, situations, and surprises that lifestyles may also have in maintain for them.

Alleviates and Eradicates Tension from the Body

The most attractive hassle of Reiki is the concept to in truth "be." The method of Reiki healing is wonderful described as a few minutes of complete rest wherein the individual receiving the strength can rid their mind of hysteria and pressure. The transfer of energy thru Reiki can make human beings experience cushty and in a few way lighter, which permits them get in touch with their inner self and promote self-reflect in their lives.

Gets Rid of Energy Blocks and Balances the Mind, Body, and Spirit

Regular Reiki treatment promotes the consistent waft of electricity within the route of the body thru getting rid of any strength blocks that may be restricting or disturbing the float of strength between the notable chakras of the body. Doing this releases the mind from pressure, enhances memory and learning abilities, and promotes intellectual readability and physical healing.

When the pathways that permit the go with the flow of strength are blocked because of stress or trauma, powerful strength is restricted from flowing into certain additives of the body—depending upon wherein the blockage is gift. This effects in mood swings, anger, fear, lack of confidence, and ache. Reiki restoration practices will let you take away the ones electricity blocks and keep those strength pathways smooth.

Gets Rid of Toxins and Improves the Immune Systems

Many Reiki restoration strategies are also used to provoke recovery with the useful resource of reminding our our our bodies to get right proper right into a mode of "self-repair" or "self-recovery," enhancing your capability to relaxation, get higher, and digest food. By triggering the body and thoughts to provoke this state, our our our bodies start to take away the terrible energies and pollutants that would in any other case be inflicting trouble or soreness. It additionally enables the frame protect itself from disorder, exhaustion, and burnout and forestalls the immune system from becoming compromised.

Improves the Quality of Sleep

Reiki durations are highly enjoyable, and that sort of rest can help your frame sleep higher, have more intellectual readability, and heal better. Do not be amazed or disappointed in case you fall asleep all through a Reiki session, as that could be a commonplace prevalence for masses humans.

Accelerates the Self-Healing Ability of the Body

Reiki power can beautify the particular bodily systems, which includes breathing, coronary coronary heart fee, circulate, blood strain, and hormone ranges. This balanced state of the body will assist it to heal from inside.

Promotes Emotional Cleansing and Spiritual Growth

When satisfactory power is transferred through the only of a type components of the mind and frame, it enables boom the receiver's mood and improves their favored perspective on lifestyles. These effective adjustments start from interior someone, this is pondered inside the alternatives they make and the mindset they could have on the outside.

Reiki Methods

Clearing the Space with Reiki

The great Reiki energy that flows through your body in some unspecified time within the destiny of a Reiki consultation can also flow through your residing vicinity or your workspace and, in doing this, may want to have profound beneficial consequences. Moreover, the Reiki remedy that you carry out on yourself or exquisite people might be advanced appreciably if your region has furthermore been cleared with the help of Reiki energy.

Other than your strength, the strength emanating from the Earth and its magnetic field can also have an impact at the balance of your dwelling area or operating vicinity. Some of the most commonplace sources of pain may be perceived the use of digital devices, while others are subtler and need a keener revel in of intuition to come across. Space clearing can be finished the use of many one-of-a-type mediums, together with essential oils, incense/sage, or particular varieties of crystals.

Doing this will be transformative and assist considerably enhance the effectiveness of a few element which you might be engaged in. Whatever method you pick out to adopt ought to be dealt with as some aspect sacred.

Centering

Before you begin your Reiki consultation, you may need to center yourself. Gassho is one of the maximum commonplace methods of centering your self—that is wherein one places every hands in a prayer function with the thumbs positioned in competition to the breastbone. Lower your head or bow down simply so your chin rests at once on pinnacle of the center hands of your arms. While seated or repute on this characteristic, recognition on your palm chakras and sense your breath shifting over your palms.

While doing this, it is herbal for some regular thoughts to wander into your mind. The high-quality aspect to do proper right right here is to understand the ones thoughts and allow them to pass in vicinity of trying to ignore them altogether. This is the building block of any meditation method. Gassho can be practiced among twenty and thirty minutes every day to clean the mind and assist you interest on the real Reiki session.

From this characteristic, slowly go with the glide your fingers until your thumbs are on the middle of the 0.33 eye to increase your intuitive powers. While you're on this function, you ought to try to speak with your internal intentions and direct yourself to the Reiki practice on the equal time as putting apart your logical thoughts in the period in-between. Focus your thoughts at the palm chakras as you experience the go together with the float of Reiki strength.

From right here, flow into your hands slowly and area them over your navel, known as the Tanden, and allow move of all the thoughts for your thoughts as you permit the top notch Reiki power drift thru your frame. The Tanden is likewise called the location of your middle, and when you have directed your interest in the path of your middle, you may feel a balance and harmony internal your body and mind.

Using the Reiki Box

A Reiki discipline is honestly what the call indicates it's far. It's a discipline used to incorporate or channel an endless reservoir of power right into a targeted area to satisfy a certain motive. The basis of the Reiki area is that Reiki strength itself is sufficient to appear something we want for our specific intentions or missions. Since it is much less tough for us to art work with some element concrete and tangible, strolling with the Reiki discipline will help you acquire this. The location can heal using particular elements of Reiki recovery and manifestation, and it could moreover be used to deliver best Reiki strength in the course of distances to more than one subjects simultaneously.

Basic Procedure

Reiki is one of the first-rate energy-restoration techniques wherein an professional practitioner of Reiki who is properly attuned can channel this immoderate brilliant life strain into the ones in dire need of it. The great detail about it's far that it turns into possible to deliver Reiki strength for the duration of prolonged distances.

Let us take a look at one of the maximum vital and commonplace strategies used to gather pinnacle effects sooner or later of healing. When completed successfully, you're sure to get keep of great benefits, hold equilibrium within the body or mind, and prosper in existence.

Using the Reiki Box

1. Find a clean discipline crafted from inexperienced materials.

2. Make certain which you clean the box earlier than the use of it to house the most notable Reiki power.

3. Draw the Reiki electricity photograph on the field—be it on the walls, base, or lid. If you're well attuned, you can moreover draw the Reiki draw close picture.

four. Place the box amongst your fingers and often direct the Reiki electricity into it. If you are new to the exercising of Reiki, you could pass over the preceding step.

five. Use paper to prepare the intention slips—quantities of paper containing descriptions of your recuperation requests or inner maximum goals.

6. Most professional Reiki masters recommend writing the ones intentions inside the present worrying as although the ones intentions have already manifested.

7. Draw the Reiki symbols on each of the aim slips and area them into the Reiki region. Close the sector.

eight. Repeat the technique of channeling Reiki power into the container for a couple of minutes each day. Make excellent that you preserve the field in a private and steady location.

nine. Keep checking the motive slips periodically to song your improvement and discard the goal slips whose cause has already been served. Make sure that you are grateful even as discarding the ones slips.

10. Repeat the whole system.

Chapter 6: Scanning The Aura

A Reiki consultation starts offevolved by means of way of figuring out imbalances in the strength and auric field of the man or woman receiving treatment. You will find out how you may experience your auric imbalances and find out such imbalances in others. You may additionally have a take a look at what the colours of the air of mystery recommend and what bodily/intellectual/emotional situations they indicate.

A Brief History of Auras

Going again to the generation of Christian Mystics of the Middle Ages, a person's charisma modified into depicted as a slight surrounding the person as portrayed with the resource of maximum artists and painters. Over the years, many scientists and researchers have attempted to seize the human air of mystery via pics strategies and super kinds of cutting-edge generation. One of the primary images emerge as fascinated with the beneficial useful resource of Nikola Tesla in 1891. According to extra trendy ideologies, auras are depicted as colored emanations and believed to surround all living beings. The charisma is a manifestation of a person's non secular, intellectual, and physical health.

Many spiritual advisors and practitioners of Reiki declare to peer the vibrations and hues that represent a person's air of mystery.

What Is an Aura

Although many people bear in mind an aura a bizarre concept, many human beings devote some of power and time to studying the this means that of auras. If you investigate the issue, you could discover many combined opinions surrounding this rather polarizing hassle. For all of the non-believers and skeptics, auras do exist. Whether you accept as true with in it or not is all about how it's far interpreted to you, and this is wherein subjects get murky.

As constant with the felony pointers of technology, all residing beings have a very unique energy that is function of them. The power that we are speakme approximately is an immediate reflected image of our u.S. Of being. Have you ever observed how someone's presence can straight away make you revel in stressful or happy without any specific cause? This is you experiencing a response to huge varieties of strength.

Scientifically speaking, an charisma is an electromagnetic location surrounding the body of any dwelling being. On a spiritual degree, it's far believed that auras correspond to the country of our chakras and the overall state of our recognition. Each charisma is fabricated from seven one in every of a type layers that correspond to one of a kind elements of our health—spiritual, intellectual, bodily, and emotional.

Let us take a look at every air of mystery layer:

Physical Aura Layer

The bodily charisma layer is installed to our regular physical health and five senses. This layer of an air of mystery gets depleted in the direction of the hours you are aware, and it rejuvenates even as we sleep and supply relaxation to our our our bodies.

Astral Aura Layer

The astral air of thriller layer is mounted to our emotional nation and saves our emotional studies and reminiscences.

Higher Aura Layer

The higher charisma layer acts as a bridge between the one of a type aura layers. The better layer moreover acts as a bridge among yours and others' well-being. This layer is in which our middle beliefs are lengthy-hooked up, which includes selflessness and compassion.

Lower Aura Layer

The decrease air of mystery layer is installed to logical capabilities and thinking patterns. Most of our waking hours are spent on this air of secrecy. The decrease layer is engaged at the same time as our minds are focused on particular responsibilities which includes running, analyzing, or wearing out any assignment to hand.

Intuitional Aura Layer

The intuitional aura layer is also known as the 1/three eye. The intuitional air of thriller layer allows you to advantage a deeper level of recognition. An man or woman's sensitivity and instinct are heightened at the intuitional air of secrecy layer.

Spiritual Aura Layer

The non secular air of secrecy layer is in that you hook up with particular human beings over topics which may be related to spirituality. Your spiritual air of mystery will growth and become stronger and brighter even as you percent, train, and engage with one of a kind people on a spiritual degree.

Absolute Aura Layer

The absolute air of mystery layer is the layer that harmonizes all of the one-of-a-type air of thriller layers. This air of mystery layer is in which all your studies are stored, and this sediment also publications you on your life's path.

Aura Colors and Their Meanings

Every layer of the human air of mystery is represented through a particular color. The way the ones auras engage with each specific shows how dynamic you're mentally, spiritually, and physical. For example, a few air of thriller layers can also moreover seem brighter because of the reality the man or woman is probably experiencing extra vibrant strength, at the equal time as other air of mystery degrees can also seem stupid if the man or woman is feeling sick or emotionally depleted. Also, a person's air of mystery varies as air of mystery sunglasses reflect in some other way counting on where a person is in existence.

The colour of a person's air of thriller can also exchange inside the direction of the day counting on their emotions, power blockages, chakra states, and the go along with the glide of energy via the frame. What you see is what is going on at that 2d. Therefore, you need to be very cautious on the identical time as analyzing particular people's auras. Some air of mystery hues and their corresponding meanings are given underneath:

1.Turquoise: Naturally prepared, dynamic character.

2.Red: Passionate and colorful persona.

three.Yellow: Joyful and intellectual.

4. Green: Natural healer having a robust reference to nature.

5. Pink: Peaceful and harmonious.

6. Murky: Mentally or bodily sick.

7. Blue: Intuitive and non secular.

8. White: Balanced and In Harmony.

How to "Read" Auras

Learning the way to read a few other individual's aura takes an entire lot of exercising. It is all about detecting the strength round a person's frame. You begin with the aid of that specialize inside the feeling a person's presence incites inside you. While taking deep breaths, take note of the exclusive sensations you experience on your body whilst you inhale and exhale. How does someone's presence make you experience? Do you feel calm, indignant, or nervous round them?

The subsequent issue to work on is enhancing your peripheral imaginative and prescient. Since we thru and massive use our primary vision maximum of the time, it is able to make the effort to boom your peripheral vision. To boom your sensitivity to at least one-of-a-kind types of mild, an remarkable technique is to attempt to recognition on a unique spot for thirty–sixty seconds.

As referred to in advance, strength constitutes the whole thing, and each living being is crafted from power. Auras are a brilliant way of knowing what the lively kingdom of a person is. To begin seeing all of the colorations of a person's charisma, have a person stand within the the front of a white wall. Make first-class which you are a few feet a ways from them and try searching through the man or woman to the wall within the decrease back of them. With sufficient exercise, you may start to see a specific colour outlining the individual's body.

The primary problem to do not forget is that you need to not reputation at the man or woman right now and try as hundreds as you could to use your peripheral imaginative and prescient to view them. You will start to see the color and slight surrounding the individual. Our air of mystery is the electricity surrounding our frame, and it additionally acts because of the truth the lens through which you may view the world. To honestly examine someone's charisma, you want to have sufficient self-awareness to differentiate between your energy and someone else's. This approach it is essential to make certain you are aware of your air of thriller and receptive sufficient to check the strength of the alternative person.

Everyone has psychic talents hidden someplace deep interior them, in spite of the truth that maximum won't apprehend it.

In truth, it is drastically believed that extra youthful children and toddlers are higher at studying auras than adults, which might also additionally provide an cause of why the mere presence of a few humans appears to disenchanted more younger kids for no obvious purpose. While this expertise may additionally furthermore decline with age, no longer whatever is retaining us again from tapping into our psychic talents later in life.

Reading auras takes quite a few exercise and staying electricity greater than anything else. There are severa carrying sports that you could try with a view to expand your functionality to take a look at and decipher auras. Depending on a person's information, one may be able to see an aura, sense an air of thriller, or maybe "concentrate" a person's aura, which varies from one individual to some other.

How to "Interpret" Auras

Seeing someone's air of thriller is one aspect; decoding it's miles a very fantastic ballgame. Human beings are complicated creatures, and our auras are similarly complex. What we project as our aura is an interplay of many stuff, consisting of our belief, research, information, personal biases, protection mechanisms, ego, cultural lenses and the manner we apprehend the area, views on spirituality, and splendid societal impacts.

When you spot every exclusive individual's air of mystery, you are looking at it through your air of secrecy, and you are looking at it thru your ideals, perceptions, and statistics. Quickly jumping to conclusions and making snap judgments isn't always a practical aspect to do, so that you should keep away from doing that. Learning the way to use your thoughts, coronary coronary heart, and soul to make accurate readings can make the effort however, do not be disheartened in case you battle to begin with.

After you've got effectively found the manner to look and interpret auras, you'll see them everywhere spherical you, be it at the purchasing center, artwork, or nearby park.

Having masses of records may also additionally make you feel tempted to percentage the whole lot you notice or look at with others. A character's air of thriller is personal, and seeing an air of thriller may be much like looking internal someone's bed room and invading their privacy. This manner which you need to only do it as soon as you have got were given their consent to achieve this.

Reiki and Scanning Auras

To check a few different character or a consumer, start the session via announcing a prayer and requesting steering to find out the specific zones in which the man or woman desires Reiki power. The subsequent step is to vicinity your non-dominant hand (left hand/right hand relying on your alternatives) about ten or twelve inches some distance from the top of your purchaser's head.

Visualize your self, putting your interest at the palm of your hand and pay close to interest to how you are feeling. Move your hand towards the pinnacle in their head at about three to 4 inches and slowly circulate your hand above the person's head and in the path in their feet on the same time as retaining the same distance among your hand and your patron. Make superb which you float your fingers very slowly and be privy to any changes in power which you is probably registering from your palm. If you revel in any adjustments inside the strength, that is a place in which your customer calls for Reiki electricity.

Energy modifications can also furthermore appear themselves as a alternate in temperature, a tingling sensation, pressure, irregularities, the feeling of being pulled, minor electric powered powered shocks, and pulsations. These adjustments can be very small, and it can be clean as a manner to influence your self that they are only a figment of your imagination. You will want to undergo in mind your self and receive as true with in the method to paintings.

When you are in the preliminary degrees of scanning, your sensitivity to essential styles of strength may not be nicely advanced, so that you want to be even greater attentive on the identical time as beginning. As you turn out to be better versed with the exercising of scanning auras, your skills will beautify, and your Reiki intervals may be greater powerful and profound.

Once you turn out to be very adept in the approach, you can discover that you can even start scanning in conjunction with your eyes and outcomes enjoy in which the character desires Reiki energy at the same time as not having to do a bargain. Master Reiki practitioners are diagnosed to see the bad strength that plagues distressed areas of the body.

When you encounter a terrible trade within the strength place or the air of thriller of an man or woman, circulate your hand up and down spherical that location until you discover a top at which you revel in the most misery. This may be as a ways as numerous toes above the person's frame, or it could be someplace that you're feeling drawn to the touch collectively together with your hands.

Most professionals advocate that the exquisite distance is spherical four or 5 inches away from the frame. When you choose out the proper distance, deliver every your fingers over the spot and channel notable Reiki electricity into that region. Reiki energy will heal the air of thriller and promote the proper flow of strength inside the physical frame, helping the organs and tissues to heal as properly.

Continue channeling tremendous Reiki power into the detected spot until you could enjoy the drift of Reiki subsiding or until that region is healed. Once you've got completed the recovery method, rescan the location and distinct regions to ensure everything is healed. If you find every different energy blockages, maintain to channel Reiki till the whole lot feels whole.

Benefits

Scanning a person's air of mystery and recuperation their electricity difficulty has numerous fitness blessings for the purpose that root cause of maximum illnesses and fitness complications lie inside the man or woman's aura. By recovery someone's air of secrecy, you may be walking on treating the purpose of the problem, thereby restoration the issues earlier than they take region themselves physical or medically. Even after a fitness hassle or a trouble has superior in a unmarried's body, someone will reply to

Reiki recuperation if the aura is rectified and stepped forward upon.

By restoration the individual's power place first, you may assist the individual to definitely receive Reiki energy greater without issue. This will allow Prana or lifestyles force to go with the flow thru the body more quite certainly. If you want to pick out scanning and Reiki remedy, you need to go along with scanning first, permitting the Reiki remedy to be greater profound and effective.

As you have got interplay with someone's air of mystery or energy place, the two of you could growth a sturdy and intimate connection. You becomes extra privy to the unique distortions in someone's air of thriller and the troubles that might be related to their air of secrecy. With extra exercise and revel in, you could moreover get more notion into their troubles and how they have been created in the first region. This can improve your ability to facilitate restoration and help your customers to a higher degree. This artwork need to be dealt with as some thing very sacred, and also you must be ever respectful of the patron and the approach. Only with kindness and the absence of judgment are you able to perform a little aspect tremendous for the people you need to assist.

How to "Feel" Auras

If you're more of a touchy character or a kinesthetic, feeling auras may be less complicated for you than seeing them. In the psychic worldwide, this ability is known as clairsentience (i.E., the capacity to revel in topics beyond the fabric realm). When feeling auras, the palms are the perfect tool to experience subtle strength adjustments and inconsistencies in a person's air of mystery. Let us have a examine a clean workout that need to help you enlarge clairsentience. To carry out this exercise, you may require a quiet place and a few free and uninterrupted time.

Start by way of being seated in a comfortable feature. You can sit down down on a chair that offers ergonomic guide collectively in conjunction with your ft firmly grounded at the floor. Keep your eyes closed and be aware about your breathing sample. Feel the air entering your body thru the nostrils, moving through your frame, and leaving it. Continue this for a hint on the identical time as to ground yourself.

While keeping your eyes closed, deliver your fingers collectively and rub your fingers swiftly for approximately twenty–thirty seconds.

Extend your arms frontward even as retaining your elbows tightly bent and your palm handling every extraordinary at approximately one foot apart.

Move your fingers closer together slowly and be aware about what you experience or enjoy in the location among your palms.

Repeat this method on the same time as slowly drawing your palms nearer and drawing them aside. Continue to acquire this even as retaining your eyes closed. If you sense any distractions, ground your self by means of manner of the usage of focusing to your breath another time. Pay interest in your breath and the air entering your body and leaving it. This may be very powerful in grounding you and stabilizing your interest.

Repeat the hand moves whilst maintaining a near eye at the one-of-a-kind sensations, emotions, visualizations, and thoughts that would begin walking through your psyche. What do you've got a have a look at all through this exercising in the vicinity amongst your fingers?

Does the feeling or feeling alternate whilst you draw your arms further apart or carry them towards each other?

The extraordinary detail approximately this exercising is that there may be now not some factor definitively accurate or wrong. What you enjoy is your unique truth, and your observations can also additionally vary relying for your perceptions and the u . S . A . Of your charisma. With time and exercising, you can enlarge a more potent clairsentience, and your ability to enjoy auras becomes higher, a lot simply so you will be capable of carry out it at the same time as keeping your eyes huge open.

Chapter 7: Self-Healing Techniques

In this chapter, you may look at self-healing techniques with hand positions; cognizance on strategies that cope with bodily signs and symptoms and symptoms, like a tightness in a tremendous a part of the body or anxiety or ache.

When you begin your journey with Reiki, you could ought to begin via running closer to on yourself earlier than you attempt to heal others. You can most effective heal others while you are emotionally and bodily healed. This will allow your body to simply receive the strength of Reiki so you can channel it. Many human beings take courses to take a look at Reiki healing, but it is viable to check it by using yourself. Any newbie can use this e-book to investigate self-restoration thru Reiki and techniques to heal others. If you locate this hard, do no longer hesitate to sign up for a route held through the usage of experts. Focus on locating the incredible way to take your journey with Reiki to the following diploma.

Connecting With the Energy of Reiki

To connect with Reiki strength, you need to advantage a higher usa of interest. In this heightened america of the us, you may have an extended popularity that you are related to the life energy flowing through the universe. This lifestyles energy want to glide results thru you. Connecting to the energy of Reiki is the simplest and vital step, which some of novices locate tough. Even in case you warfare to attain this heightened kingdom, do not get discouraged. For people who workout meditation often or have experience in meditation, it could be plenty easier to carry out this number one step.

Connecting to the energy of the universe will contain steps. One is that you need to permit flow into of any ego and open your self to the understanding and the electricity flowing thru the universe. When you allow yourself to be an open conduit for this strength, you may attempt visualizing the go with the go with the flow of the strength through you.

You will connect to the universe's interest at the same time as to procure the country of thoughts, which allows you connect with Reiki power. For Reiki invocation, you in reality have to speak to the universe and are seeking out permission to apply its strength for recovery. You need to be calm and function readability to your thoughts at the identical time as talking to the universe. To achieve this u.S.A. Of america of mind, try meditating for a couple of minutes in advance than a Reiki invocation. It will help you loosen up and increase your functionality to connect with the awareness of the universe.

As a novice, you could pick out to talk out loud or silently on the identical time as you do all this. You can ask the universe to attach you to its electricity in any manner you want. Your private beliefs will normally manual you to choose out a selected way. The common purpose want to normally be that you may heal in a natural holistic way with unconditional love.

Take some time to decide the way you want to speak to the universe and what you want to say. Then sit down down in a quiet area and region your hands together. Your fingers have to be positioned in a prayer role inside the front of the coronary coronary heart chakra. Healing desires to go back returned from an area of love; that is why the coronary heart chakra is appropriate. Once you are prepared in this feature, you could say some element like this:

"I am calling out to the power of the universe and that of each Reiki conduit from the beyond, present, and destiny to participate on this session of healing. I name upon all the energies to help me create a strong connection with the electricity of the universe. I ask for the infinite popularity a superb way to equip me to channel this ordinary electricity. I ask that the same antique power flows via all of me and that I can use its power to behavior herbal and loving recuperation. I ask for the data that lets in you to assist me use and channel this power inside the outstanding way feasible. I ask for empowerment from the divine love and advantages of the universe."

Asking for permission from the universe is vital for Reiki recovery. Do now not awareness on yourself or have an ego that makes you determined which you are completely able to restoration. You should be steady with the power of the universe for it to waft via your frame so that you can act as a channel for recuperation. Your popularity need to be better, and your vibrational energy desires to be extended.

Pay interest to the manner you speak and ask for permission to emerge as a conduit. It manner that you'll be soliciting for permission to grow to be a conductor of the attention and information of the universe in preference to asking to emerge as a healer or making choices on your very own. This will handiest be viable in case you allow circulate of your ego and allow your beliefs to be aligned with the consciousness of the universe.

Universal electricity is not seen to the naked eye as it exists past the physical realm. This is why you could connect with it first-class if your thoughts is in a heightened kingdom of recognition. To "see" it, you want to visualise. Visualization will help you experience a physical connection with the energy of the universe. Close your eyes and take a deep breath in.

When you let move of this breath, recollect some blue-white colored electricity beams surrounding you. Visualize the ones beams like threads stretching from the floor to the sky and into the rest of the universe. You will be able to experience this energy as you visualize. Then take every exclusive breath in. While letting a deep breath out, interest the strength in your arms, and speak out to the everyday strength. When you breathe, take the infinite light in and speak to for it in your palms as you visualize the energy coming into internal your body.

While the electricity flows thru your frame and out from your hands, visualize the cool white strength sparkling to your hands. As you try this, you'll experience the electricity of the universe as it radiates through your arms.

When you hire the device of visualization, you ought to keep in mind that it does not depend what you believe the power as. You can don't forget it in any color or shape. The purpose is for it that will help you revel in that power. It doesn't count number wide variety if you can't see the strength. What subjects is your willingness and energy of will to hook up with it. You might be able to heal with the universe's power whilst your mind and will are aligned so that you can act as a conduit.

Scanning the Aura

Most humans have an incorrect notion of ways auras exist. Your air of thriller isn't always a few visible power or some issue that your frame creates. Aura is, in reality, the electricity of the universe. It is the strength surrounding each residing aspect and isn't always simply "around" them like many humans recollect. A person's air of mystery exists within the frame, too, so it's now not honestly projected outward. Your air of mystery is a part of the electricity system in you. It works due to the fact the thoughts because it takes in and places out records. It can get hold of and transmit indicators from the location spherical you.

The fitness of your air of thriller is determined with the aid of manner of the whole lot inner you. This is why your charisma can also appear to be a darkish blob if you have many terrible mind. We have already described that auras can have unique colorings as they transmit records approximately your body and thoughts. They also can have numerous shapes, sizes, styles, or textures. Your aura isn't always continually a stable coloration. When there are discolorations, or there can be texture, there is probably versions in colorations.

When someone connects to the strength of the universe, they are able to sense the strength round them. If you want to visualise this electricity, close to your eyes, and region your arms simply above your head. Keep your fingers coping with toward your body. You can use each of your fingers or your dominant hand for this exercising. While defensive your hands up on this position, hold them approximately 3–six inches far from your frame.

Chapter 8: Reiki

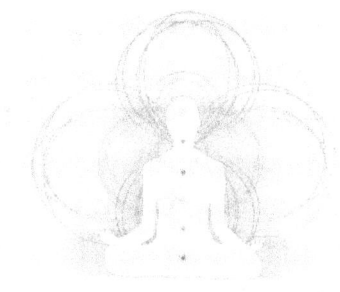

Reiki is break up into branches: Japanese Reiki and Western Reiki.

The Fundamentals

In popular, there are 3 levels of understanding: first, 2nd, and 1/3 degree. Those who exercise reiki is probably capable of heal and treatment themselves in addition to others.

Distance healing is a term used to offer an reason behind the ability of the second diploma of practitioners to treatment and heal everybody from afar. The most degree (the most advanced) is the important level at which the practitioner is meticulously informed and proficient in case you want to edify and attune others to reiki exercise.

In smooth phrases, it's miles a clean recovery idea primarily based mostly on holistic techniques and with out the use of any medicinal drugs. The practitioner performs the method through setting his or her palms on the individual that requires recovery.

The essential concept inside the back of the method is for the practitioner to deliver incredible electricity to the recipient at the identical time as attractive within the recovery way. Some normal claims had been made, claiming that recovery energy is self-looking for and might "zero in" at the wound to start the healing way.

The powerful electricity that is supposed to be emitted for curing and restoration features is the most brilliant characteristic of the reiki recovery method. Because the practitioner's electricity is stated to be excessive best and at most appropriate ranges, she or he ought to adhere to high-quality practices so you may be a a achievement practitioner. Keeping the frame and mind as smooth and natural as possible is one of the most critical elements.

The majority of people however agree with that Japanese reiki focuses extra on specific regions that need restoration, in region of the second kind of western reiki, which treats the entire frame.

Chapter 9: Learning Approximately Reiki

Although Reiki has been round for a long term, it is best on this era that it is being considered as an opportunity to standard and ultra-modern medical remedies. Learning and acquiring facts on this form of art work is straightforward and does no longer necessitate large education, nor does analyzing it necessitate or take some years. The splendor of reiki is how easily it can be handed from trainer to pupil with out inflicting bias.

Getting Schooled

As energy is transferred from one frame to every other for recuperation functions, a easy and natural thoughts set is wanted to be a successful reiki practitioner.

To be a a fulfillment practitioner, you want to have this sort of exceptional strength. Some human beings agree with that the reiki healing way is just like God's recovery strategies, at the same time as others agree with that the thoughts and body are related.

Several human beings who've taken this shape of paintings drastically and characteristic verified psychic records. Many others believe they have got heightened focus of their environment and own "0.33 eye" abilities.

The exercise is totally targeted on one's very own non-public fitness troubles and the manner to treatment them. The functionality to attach first-rate energy from one body to some different aids inside the recuperation of health problems.

This recuperation way has been a achievement in the palms of numerous human beings. These are folks that refuse to comply with the western clinical way. This reiki secret is easy to investigate and could live with you for the relaxation of your lifestyles. The method is difficult to overlook.

The a success reiki workout has an impact on the man or woman's complete body, mind, and emotions. Toxins gather in our structures over the years, causing negativity within the body, but reiki permits to smooth the negativity and bring in exceptional energy.

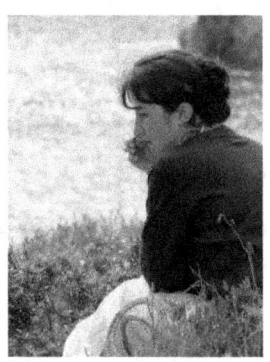

Chapter 10: Negative Effects And Sides Of Reiki

There are generally incredible and bad elements to the whole thing in lifestyles. Reiki follows the equal pattern. It takes time and effort to make the selection to start the method of reading reiki. A high-quality level of dedication and perseverance is anticipated, which may be hard to control in present day society of "immediately gratification" expectations.

What To Look For

To make certain that a potential reiki practitioner is capable of attracting extremely good power, she or he want to make a few lifestyles sacrifices. The first step is to abstain from ingesting non-vegetarian components for a few days earlier than beginning reiki.

Consuming non-vegetarian food, drinks containing pollutants, alcohol, capsules, pesticides, and other risky materials want to be averted even as working inside the course of reiki. These negative elements throw the machine off balance and make it tough for amazing electricity to go with the flow smoothly.

A liquid juice weight-reduction plan is the handiest method. It is likewise critical to lessen or get rid of the consumption of pollution. These factors purpose discord within the worried device in addition to the endocrine device. Alcohol, candies, and smoking are some more things to keep away from as a minimum three days in advance than performing a reiki session.

Maintaining a relaxed and quiet lifestyle is also beneficial, but with current annoying life, this could be hard. Similarly, proscribing your exposure to bad outside influences is critical; therefore, searching television, paying attention to horrifying tune, and analyzing frightening data ought to all be avoided.

Aside from the terrible elements mentioned above, it's also critical to avoid worry, anger, jealousy, fear, and hate.

These feelings might also need to make it tough for someone to come to be a a hit reiki practitioner and to conduct reiki commands.

In a few intense times, reiki practitioners are trying to find to isolate themselves from others genuinely because they trust and consider that the ones round them are impure with bad energy with which they do not want to be associated.

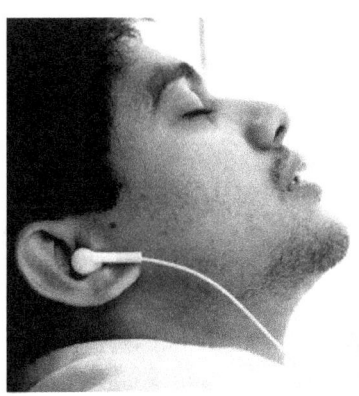

Chapter 11: Taking Reiki Into Consideration For Health Benefits

It's easy to feel uneasy whilst you have a look at that a person has a scientific situation. The primary supply of hysteria is the complex medical strategies that want to be lengthy long gone via on the same time as already in a precarious state of affairs. Furthermore, having to pick out the various numerous remedy options to be had for the aforementioned medical health situations may be tough to say the least.

A Mind Opener

People are interested in exploring restoration strategies at the same time as easy and clean strategies are available to get over health troubles. Similarly, ignoring the winning treatment for the scientific situation and tactics, the reiki method of treatment is not an choice to recollect. To positioned it a few different way, reiki want to no longer be carried out in location of different ongoing scientific treatments.

Reiki is a holistic treatment this is meant to complement any preexisting remedy the affected character can be receiving at the outset.

The reiki issue is supposed to art work with first rate energy in case you want to combat any preexisting negatives in the person's machine. Because reiki electricity is supposed to be remoted primarily based totally on the specific place in need of excellent energy.

After incorporating reiki as a complementary restoration device, human beings tormented by excessive clinical situations have noted a high charge of achievement.

The effective electricity despatched to the character affected by the scientific state of affairs by using way of the person acting reiki is regularly described as calming and useful. This remarkable power flows thru his or her body, and most of his or her illnesses may be alleviated to 3 degree. There is likewise the possibility of without a doubt disposing of the ailment if the exercising is sustained for a long time.

Those who take their health with no consideration and do not take precautions to preserve a healthy weight loss program and way of life can also benefit from analyzing reiki to gain a better understanding of the significance of authentic bodily and intellectual health.

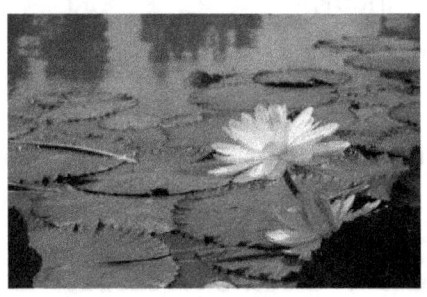

Chapter 12: Reiki To Solve Problems In Life

The majority of people who've had some experience with the reiki global of awesome power praise it. Most human beings be given as true with it is a form of artwork that the complete worldwide can advantage from, regardless of the fact that it's far marketed as an effective and calming exercise.

The Advantages

Most bodily and highbrow illnesses, similarly to environmental cruelty, were connected to lousy factors in a few unspecified time inside the destiny. Reiki can assist to take away some of this poor energy and update it with the satisfactory first-rate energy.

Reiki is a way that addresses the mind, body, and environment, all of which might be related in some way. The factors of the mind, consisting of the questioning manner, can be tuned to have most effective first-rate mind even as reiki is used to address the mind.

Many accurate subjects may be completed and even spill over into your environment on the same time as the thoughts is educated to be tremendous all the time. Aside from the idea technique, the reiki fashion of transmitting brilliant power from one person to a few other can aid in the improvement of a higher highbrow u . S .. Migraines, complications, stress, worry, and quite some tremendous mind-related conditions can be effectively handled with the awesome energy received through reiki exercising.

This immoderate exceptional reiki electricity is in popular used to do away with all bad power that reasons or contributes to the person's sickness.

One of the most first-rate advantages of the way is that it's miles painless. In fact, the majority of people who have attested to experiencing a comforting higher feeling and in some cases provide extremely good relaxation and snoozing off inside the path of a session are common.

The reiki recuperation technique additionally may be completed from afar. This unusual feature is a bonus for the ones looking for this form of healing to supplement their current-day scientific remedy. A expert reiki practitioner can results and quietly transfer pleasant strength via quiet meditation.

Chapter 13: More Benefits Of Reiki

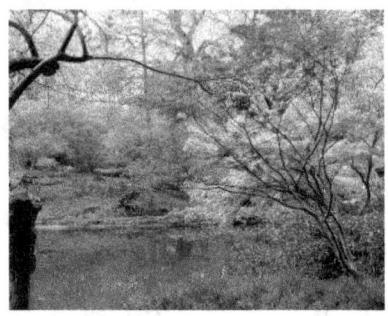

Reiki is one of the oldest and maximum historical strategies of moving superb electricity from one source to a few other for the cause of recovery.

The reiki workout has numerous advantages within the practitioner's life. Reprieve from highbrow and physical pressure, consolation in frame and mind, relaxation, and peace inside the environment are a number of the extra famous and common benefits obtained via working towards reiki.

A Few More Benefits

There are a slew of various famous reiki blessings, none of which might be any a lot much less beneficial. The majority of practitioners exercise so you can advantage non secular readability.

Reiki assists within the remedy of emotional sorrow and misery thru the use of connecting one to a few different thru the middle of 1's spirituality, preventing the thoughts and body from turning into absolutely tired.

Reiki additionally allows to relieve ache at the identical time as furthermore enhancing blood pass all through the body. Reiki can also assist to rush up the healing of youngster bleeding wounds via doing so. A form of reiki practitioners additionally attest to the blessings of reiki's purification detail within the arteries, gall bladder, liver, lungs, and spleen.

Many specific diseases have been dealt with and cured with reiki, that is taken into consideration a complementary remedy to modern scientific treatments and medicinal pills.

Reiki has been used to make high-quality changes in the wounded vicinity for severa clinical situations which may be normally connected to 3 sort of unevenness. Few medical conditions, collectively with persistent and acute nostril bleeds, despair, and chronic insomnia, have placed reiki to be fairly useful in their recovery.

Reiki is also identified to hasten the restoration device, particularly after surgical strategies. Positive power transfer aids in hastening a brilliant healing without the usage of more medicines.

Chapter 14: Using Reiki Effectively

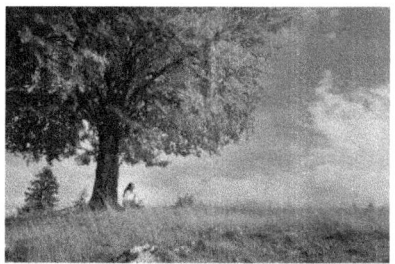

When someone is undergoing treatment for a clinical state of affairs, he or she is likewise exposed to some of terrible elements.

The bad necessities introduced because of gift remedies might also increase the person's bodily and intellectual stress, resulting in an entire lot of different headaches and a slower healing price.

Putting It Into Action

Various humans have said elevated restoration prices and remarkable strength after combining reiki healing with medical remedy for their clinical conditions.

These adjustments propose that the individual's fitness has advanced because of the exercising. Furthermore, the powerful strength reduces remedy use via rushing up recovery.

Before searching ahead to exceptional results and changes, reiki need to be practiced for a splendid amount of time. Changes in exceptional areas, which includes new highbrow capabilities introduced on through the effective electricity, additionally may be felt this way.

The workout of shifting high-quality strength should be finished with the recipient's cooperation and willingness to find out this fashion of recovery so one can gain from reiki correctly. A fine intellectual attitude is essential for accomplishing reiki achievement.

Several scientific researchers well known the strength of immoderate first-class energy, especially on the equal time as it is used for recuperation. Scientists are notoriously skeptical, so this kind of acknowledgement proves that reiki can be a useful device within the restoration approach. Most scientists even accept as actual with that the exquisite element is truly determined in anybody, and that studying to control this power has good sized fitness benefits.

The excellent way to discover ways to use reiki for recovery or to advantage a holistically wholesome frame and mind is to undergo the technique yourself. Because there are not any recognized issue consequences, reiki is a hazard-unfastened exercise.

Chapter 15: Additional Treatment Advantages Of Reiki

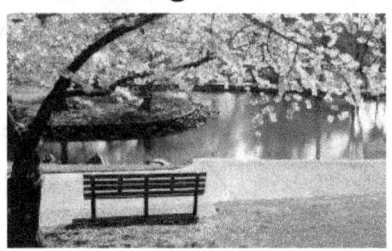

In the scientific discipline, new discoveries are made each day. Some are upbeat, on the equal time as others are not. Others can be prohibitively expensive to recall, so whilst a leap forward like reiki is made, it is able to be a boon to the ones in want of this shape of promising treatment.

Additional Discoveries

Despite the truth that reiki has been round for a long term and has been successfully practiced in hundreds of ancient cultures, typically Asian, it's far unexpectedly gaining reputation a number of the more youthful technology.

With first-rate effects, a few athletes have chosen to apply this approach of recuperation to complement their ongoing clinical treatments.

Many athletes' healing strategies have prolonged because of using the superb strength that reiki style of treatment is based totally absolutely mostly on to counteract the horrible factors of an harm.

The fact that the affected vicinity is in "higher than earlier than" scenario presents to the pretty short healing time.

With the usage of reiki in regions where Aids has brought about untold misery for masses people, a few new breakthroughs have moreover been made.

This promising u . S . A . Of the usage of reiki as a wonderful power to combat all the poor results of Aids is attractive many human beings to strive it out.

Another powerful way of healing an illness is thru distance recuperation using the reiki technique. Because it is not usually feasible or convenient to be via a affected man or woman's facet for numerous reasons, reiki isn't only drastically used however moreover touted to be genuinely as powerful in presenting heaps-wanted comfort and recuperation.

Some human beings who've been practising reiki for a long time have even been documented as selling this form of recovery for animals.

Some humans have have become to reiki for its non-invasive and mild fashion of remedy while seeking out the excellent treatment for his or her appreciated puppy. There have been numerous evaluations of fulfillment due to the fact this technique does no longer upload to the strain of an already sick pup.

Chapter 16: What To Expect From Reiki Practice

If you're considering attempting reiki for the number one time, it is a great idea to research as an lousy lot as you could about the art work shape first.

Things To Consider

Some of the areas recommended for studies earlier than making relevant options including in which, whilst, and who to touch are as follows:

Reiki's blessings

The approach for remedy

Reiki certification

If there are any remedy fees, what are they?

Reiki education

Reiki demonstrations and testimonials

Reiki practitioners with a great recognition

Materials and gear that might be used

When task critical studies, preserve in mind that surfing the net for precise necessities takes time and patience. There is lots of statistics to be had near reiki, and a number of it is pretty contradictory.

The inconsistency stems from the numerous mind and philosophies which is probably concerned in the test and workout of this artwork shape. The numerous testimonials to be had will assist you to make an informed preference, no matter the reality that they may be complicated at instances.

It's additionally a first-rate concept to apply the internet to find the nearest appropriate reiki center, agency, or society. Several studying substances also are to be had to analyze more approximately the reiki restoration artwork shape and holistic approach to the frame and thoughts.

It have to be said, however, that this unique artwork shape may be quite individualistic at instances. Many human beings have used reiki on themselves with terrific fulfillment.

The reiki fashion permits you to apply this artwork shape to address your body and mind even as no longer having to be near a healer. Individually, Reiki may be used to create a fantastic surroundings for amusement and comfort in one's very personal privacy.

Chapter 17: Drawbacks Of Not Using Reiki

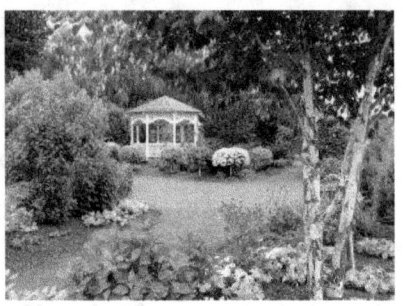

Today, nearly all illnesses or ailments necessitate invasive scientific remedy. When someone discovers the presence of a possible negative fitness situation, their anxiety levels are high-quality to be driven to their limits.

As a end result, any non-invasive possibility or complementary treatment or remedy can be very reassuring.

What You Could Be Missing

Reiki gives the critical leverage to combat a bad state of health this is causing or has introduced approximately the presence of a sickness because of the reality it is a workout of shifting awesome electricity proper right into a terrible surroundings.

There is a huge lack of capability recovery or arrest of the medical situation if the possibility of using reiki for treatment of fitness conditions isn't always explored.

Reiki now not quality aids in physical restoration, however it moreover aids inside the highbrow country of mind.

Many scientific troubles seem to start or be attributed to an person's united states of the usa of mind, so the use of reiki because step one in stopping the ailment or contamination can start.

Because reiki may be used on oneself, it may be used on a regular foundation to promote a brilliant outlook in lifestyles. With a higher mental kingdom of mind that contributes to a powerful outlook, the character's excellent of lifestyles can be highly profitable.

Although there hasn't been plenty research completed to provide conclusive evidence, a few sources have attested to the general awesome revel in whilst reiki is used during being pregnant. This end is based completely clearly on the reality that reiki practitioners have hundreds of superb power in their our bodies and minds. The scenario and nicely-being of the infant also are confident because of the stated extremely good energy that surrounds the expectant mom. The exercising of reiki has a nice issue impact of happier and healthier toddlers.

www.ingramcontent.com/pod-product-compliance
Lightning Source LLC
Chambersburg PA
CBHW071446080526
44587CB00014B/2010